ABOUT THE AUTHOR:

Edward Obaidey graduated from the Tokyo Therapeutic Institute in 1990, and has a busy practice in Tokyo. He is the founder of the Japanese Acupuncture and Moxibustion Skills Foundation, an organisation dedicated to the practice and preservation of traditional Oriental Medicine, and has given seminars in England, Australia, Canada, Japan and America. He is privileged to have studied in apprenticeship under *Misao Takenouchi sensei* and with his current teacher, *Masakazu Ikeda sensei* for whom he has assisted in the presentation of many seminars abroad. In keeping with his traditional training, Mr. Obaidey's clinic is a centre both of healing, and of the continuous learning and development of his students, visitors and himself.

Edward Obaidey translated *"The Practice of Japanese Acupuncture and Moxibustion: Classic Principles in Action"* (Eastland Press; ISBN: 0-939616-43-2) by *Masakazu Ikeda sensei*. This text is highly recommended as an in-depth introduction to classical acupuncture in Japan. The only other of *Ikeda sensei's* many books currently available in English (also recommended) is *"Integration of Acupuncture and Herbal Medicine: Theory and Practice"* (ISBN: 978-0-578-06534-2)

A LONG ROAD

an acupuncture travelogue   vol. I

edward obaidey

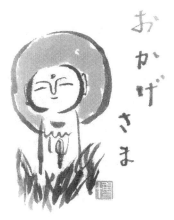

おかげさま

A LONG ROAD

an acupuncture travelogue   vol. I

Cover Illustration by *Hiroshi Ando*. He has drawn a *Jizou-sama* which is a Buddhist figurine found in local districts. It embodies his feeling concerning the term "*Okagesama*" written in Japanese hiragana as "おか げさま" (お蔭様 in *Kanji*). This is a statement of intent towards the whole process of life and living. It is an expression of universal thanks based on the understanding that one's very existence is dependent quite considerably on the good will of others.

The author feels very fortunate to have *Hiroshi Ando* as his father in law.

Okagesama de!

Cover Design by Benigna Iwasaki
Interior Illustrations by Yuka Obaidey; formatted by John Blazevic
Book Design & Editing by Toby Stephens

Volume I

A Long Road will be published in a number of Volumes. Material for Volume II and Volume III will include the following, although slight variations may be made at time of printing.
If you would like to be informed when Volume II, Volume III and any further Volumes or other publications by the author are available, please send an e-mail with the words "Long Road" as the subject to rareapricotpress@gmail.com.

Volume II

Volume III

Figures

Tables

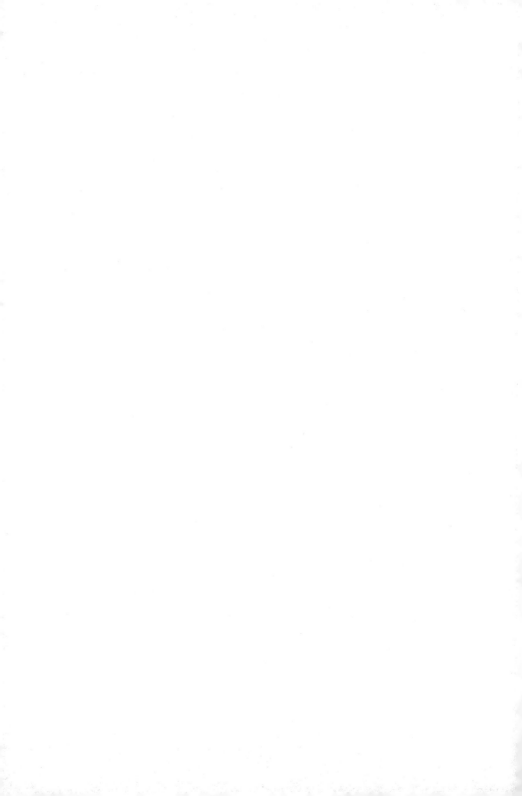

Foreword

- by Ikeda Masakazu Sensei -

エドワード・オベイディー氏と出会ったのは２０年も前のことだ。確か、京都で学会があったときに私の実技を見て興味を持ったらしい。後で聞くと、実技の内容ではなく、その賑やかな performance が良かったという。鍼灸師は陰気な人が多いのに私だけは異質だったらしい。

数年後、彼の発案でオーストラリアでセミナーを開くことになった。もちろん彼が通訳をしてくれた。その後、オーストラリアはもちろんのこと、アメリカでのセミナーも彼が通訳してくれた。もう２０回ちかくもお世話になっている。

彼の通訳を聞いた人は解ると思うが、私とのやりとりは喜劇役者同士の間の取り方に似ている。だから講演の間は爆笑が絶えない。日本語と英語の両方が解る人にとってはさらに面白いという。私のジョークを更に面白くして彼が話するからである。

断っておくが、講演がジョークの連続だというわけではない。たとえば何かの質問があって私が答えると、彼は私の言ったことを、そのまま通訳することは少ない。彼自身が理解していることを交えて通訳している。言い換えると、私の講演だけど、半分近くは彼が講演していると言ってもよい。私は、これは実にすばらしいことだと思っている。受講生は非常に理解しやすいからである。これはしかし、簡単なことではない。彼自身が中国の古典医術あるいは日本の伝統医術を理解しているからできることである。

欧米はキリスト教文化である。これは個人の自立を尊ぶ。つまり個人としての意見をしっかりと持つように教育される。これは非常に大切なことで、日本人には欠落している部分である。しかし、

その自立が悪く出ると利己主義になり、他人の意見を聴かなくなる。それはそれで良いのだが、伝統を学ぶとなれば話は変わってくる。自分の意見は棄てて最初から学ばないと体得できないのが伝統医術である。その点、エドワード氏は、まるで日本の昔ながらの徒弟制度で鍛えられたような柔軟さと奥深さを持っている。

オーストラリアやアメリカでは一人の先生の名前を冠して◎◎スタイルなどという。しかし、彼の理論や実技は決してエドワードスタイルではない。もし言うのであればTJMスタイルであろうか。

本書は、その一部を記したものだが、日本の伝統医術を理解するのが難しい欧米の人たちにとっては朗報であろう。一人でも多くの人が本書を繙き、臨床に応用されることを願って序文とする。

経絡治療学会学術部長
池田政一

- Translation[1] of Foreword -

I first met Edward Obaidey over 20 years ago at an acupuncture conference in Kyoto. He came to my clinical demonstration and showed great interest in it. Later I heard it was not the actual content of the demonstration that impressed him but my exuberant performance of it. Apparently so many of the other acupuncturists were gloomy and somber types that this was radically different, and I really stood out.

Several years later, acting on his idea, I held an acupuncture seminar in Australia. He, of course, was my translator. Since then there have been numerous seminars in Australia and the United States where he has served as my translator. We have given about 20 seminars together.

People who have heard his translation will probably know what I mean

---

[1] Translation by Charles Homonnay

when I say that we interact like 2 vaudeville comedians on stage. Throughout the lecture the audience repeatedly bursts into boisterous laughter. The audience members who know both Japanese and English seem to laugh even harder. The reason is because when I say something funny in Japanese he expands it and makes it even better in English.

However, do not take this to mean that the lecture is just one joke after another. Let's take the case of a question to which I answer. He rarely translates what I say word for word. He translates what I say with his additional understanding. So, while it is my presentation, it is fair to say he contributes almost an additional 50%. I think this is wonderful because the participants really can get a good understanding. This superior translation is not an easy feat. It is possible because Edward Obaidey truly understands the ancient Chinese medical classics as well as the practice of traditional Japanese medicine.

European/western culture has deep roots in the Judeo-Christian tradition. Part of this manifests as respect for the individual. People are brought up to have their own individual views. I believe this is important, and I can see how a lack of this adversely affects many Japanese people. However, this individuality and independence also can lead in a bad direction to self-centeredness in which people are not able to listen to the views of others. This may even be acceptable sometimes, but when it comes to learning a traditional art with a deep context it is a different matter. Unless you can discard your individual views and attachments and learn from a new beginning with a clear mind you cannot master the art of traditional medicine. It is this level of flexibility and deep understanding that Edward Obaidey has attained by going through the traditional apprentice system, just as if it were in the Japan of long ago.

In Australia and America people sometimes take the name of an individual practitioner and elevate it to a style of therapy: So-and-so style of acupuncture. However this man's knowledge and skill is absolutely not "Edward style." If you had to put a name to it maybe you could call it "traditional Japanese medicine" (TJM style).

This book presents a piece of the tradition, but to people in the English speaking world for whom it is difficult to understand this traditional medicine this book is good news. I wrote this introduction with the hope that people will read this book and apply it to their clinical practice.

Masakazu Ikeda,
Meridian Therapy Association Academic Chairman

Introduction

It is rather strange to see all of this on paper. Some of it is familiar but quite a lot of it is somewhat foreign to me. The reason for this is that this book represents snap shots of what I thought, said or did at different periods of my development. Some of it now appears rather basic to me at this time but it seems that I felt strongly enough to write about it at the time. I must make it clear that quite a few of the treatment methods and approaches I no longer use now.

When I was a student at school, struggling through my text books in Japanese, I used to love reading about individual practitioners and the methods that they developed to help their patients. Some of the books were written in a manner that allowed me to feel I was standing right next to them when they performed their treatments. When I read these books, any weariness that I may have had just melted away and I really enjoyed it. I read about Japanese, Korean, Chinese practitioners of oriental medicine but also practitioners of Osteopathic and Chiropractic medicine, Shamanic healing practices and *Qi Gong* self healing episodes. All of these various books that I read took healing from theory into reality via my imagination as I read their stories. The constant was the individual and the efforts they put forth in their art. This touched my heart and made me want to follow a good teacher and one day become like them.

All of this that you have in front of you originated from my teachers and was merely expressed through me at a certain time in a certain place.

I give great thanks to my teacher *Masakazu Ikeda Sensei* who has been so generous with his knowledge, skill and time. It is no exaggeration to say that he has opened up a whole new world for myself and patients. Words will always be insufficient to express my gratitude.

A big thanks to John Blazevic who began what must have been the truly uniquely boring task of compiling.

Most credit though must go to Toby Stephens whose dogged determination was able to make a book out of this with the almost complete non co-operation of the author. In other words, me. Well done Toby, for once your stubbornness has borne edible fruit.

Lastly I must never forget my poor patients who have put up with me for so many years and still retain a sense of humour even in the midst of sometimes terminal disease. To you I make this pledge: ***I promise I will be a little better than I was yesterday but not quite as good as I will be tomorrow.***

Edward Obaidey, Tokyo 2011

FUNDAMENTALS

Note: These fundamental tenets are all considered to be of equal importance and are therefore all numbered "1".

1 Respect the Teachings

The body of Oriental medicine left to us by the ancients was written at a time when there were no lecture circuits, seminars or schools. In other words profit was not a motive of concern for the authors. They were written for the benefit of mankind. As such they are very precious and deserve respect.

1 Respect the Teacher

The teacher embodies the teachings and therefore should be respected for their skill, knowledge and experience. If the student does not respect the teacher then it is a defective relationship that can achieve very little. The teacher will be unable to pass on anything meaningful and the student will be closed to real knowledge.

1 Put the Patient First

Too often practitioners will give this lip service but while treating, the main concern is often themselves. On a physical level, I have noticed that when I am treating people, people observing or even assisting me, may start to massage themselves or stretch their tight areas. This signifies a fundamental misunderstanding of the treatment process and that their *Ki* is not concentrated where it should be.

1 Be Humble

If you already know it all, then there is nothing more to learn. I have never met anyone like this but it is a possibility. If you do not know everything and wish to learn, then being humble is the best way to learn. Instead of making a point of telling everybody how much you know, how about keeping quiet and letting the teacher teach you what they know? It is far more efficient and satisfying.

1 Constantly Strive

Always try to give your best in your treatments, study and dealings with fellow human beings.

SU WEN & LING SHU REFERENCES

All classical references to the *Ling Shu* (Spiritual Pivot) and the *Su Wen* (Simple Questions) are based on the translation into Japanese by *Yasuzo Shibasaki* (柴崎保三). My preference for his work entitled "Acupuncture and Moxibustion Medicine Compendium *Su Wen Ling Shu* (鍼灸医学大系 黄帝內経素問霊枢)" published by *Yu Kon Sha* (雄渾社) in 1980 is for both personal and academic reasons.

During my second year in acupuncture school in Tokyo, I was fortunate enough to be a member of *Shibasaki Sensei's* study group. Unfortunately he was already old and frail and I never got to study under him personally but through his number one student *Nakajima Sensei*, I became somewhat familiar with the direction of his life's work. I also remember making preparations with other members of the study group for his funeral when *Shibasaki Sensei* passed away. At the funeral there were various wreaths from all over Japan and also even from abroad. But I noticed with great sadness that there was no wreath from the school that he graduated from and that I was at that time studying at. I thought that this was a disgrace and I vowed at that time that I would make sure that his name was not forgotten.

The second reason is that the rigour and sheer bloody mindedness of his work just cannot be ignored. He spent around 25 years of his life working on a detailed translation of the Yellow Emperor's Internal Classic based on a sound breakdown of the meaning of the Chinese characters at the time they were written. This was achieved through a personal relationship with the top authority in the field at the time from Tokyo university. He was a military man on a passionate mission and approached his monumental task with military like precision and no compromises. The result was a series of volumes which have now long been out of print.

When I graduated from acupuncture school I spent an arm and a leg getting hold of these volumes and it gives me great pleasure to use them for the purpose that they were written for - to illuminate the ancient wisdom for those in need in the present.

CHAPTER 1

General

1.1   GENERALISATION

It is generalisation and the application of its principles that lead to the best results. Even specific measures and modalitites are useful in as much as they restore general function. Bear in mind that the hallowed Oriental medical philosophies such as that of Heaven Man and Earth (天地人) are also principles of generality ("POG").

"Specialist" is a term that encourages trust and a belief that good or better than normal ("special") results will be obtained. However, often the reverse is true. The specialist is often hampered by "tunnel vision" and thus may make unwise decisions.

The true oriental medical practitioner is a "specialist in generality". The tendancy to specialise is unfortunately another manifestation of "looking for a short-cut" and the "grasping mentality of the mind".

The application of generality in one's daily life is a type of enlightenment. On the train whilst travelling toward your destination you will better appreciate the view, the sky, the sunshine, the shadows on your lap.

In more specific examples, the same is true. Application of general principles (letting go of the goal orientated mentality) results in better form which must in turn lead to better results. At this stage the goal specific mentality can be introduced as an energy source but never at the expense of the general principles.

Thus in *Tai Chi*, movement is not the goal. Rather it is the result. If movement were the goal, then after learning and remembering a number of set movements the study would be complete. This is however not the case. Instead of the person demonstrating movement with their built-in faults intact, we target the faults by means of general principles. It is when these principles are applied that the movement becomes perfect. In the case of *Tai Chi* the principles are so profound that their correct application will automatically mean great health, peace of mind, longevity and extremely satisfactory fighting prowess. Unfortunately if any of these attributes becomes the focus, this "specificness" will greatly intefere with the "generality" of the principles and thus lead to reduced results. This is especially true of fighting prowess which if introduced as a goal early on, will severly hamper ones progress.

Perhaps the ultimate display of *Tai Chi* principles can be seen in the standing meditation. This is where movement is completely taken out of the equation leaving only the general principles to discipline the body and mind. This curious exercise has produced people with serious fighting ability, power and grace, amongst them my teacher Tam Sam *Sifu* (師父).

In social interaction as well, generality and its application will lead to generosity in a very natural way. An appreciation of the predicament of one's fellow man and one's own part in it is a natual consequence of generality. In business the urge to sell is tempered by a wider vision including that of the buyer, leading to greater understanding of consumer demand. Consistent application of generality will lead to a gradual cessation of shortsighted, short term profit oriented business practice. Instead, holistic long-term business practice where the relationship between buyer and seller rather than the sales figures will again be restored to its rightful place.

This will lead to trust and confidence which, at the end of the day, drives all financial markets and business. Over time this must also lead to better use of resources and a natural inclination toward sustainability.

Now as you can see, I think I have made the case quite clearly and strongly for generalisation. But still when we approach treatment we have to be extra vigilant not to lose these principles. The patient, after all, most commonly presents with a specific complaint and whilst suffering from this disease is in no position to view things in generalist terms. Indeed, we can say that in many cases it is a lack of generality that predisposes them to disease in the first place.

As practitioners it is important that we apply the principles of generality ("POG") to allow us to experience empathy with the patient as well as to see the big picture. This can be distinguished from over-identification with the patient to the extent that the POG are lost. When this occurs the patient and the practitioner will find that they both inhabit a dark narrow hole burrowed deep by tunnel vision. This is especially prevalent when there is an emotional attachment between the patient and practitioner.**

No, the patient and their suffering must be illuminated by application of the POG so that correct treatment and a genuine sense of compassion is evoked resulting in a cure.

Genuine treatment then, is the result of applying the POG to remedy an ailment whether it be specific or not. The hallmark of genuinely low level treatment is the application of specific principles to a specific illness resulting not in a cure but a more serious general disease.

** I am reminded at this point of an incident that occurred in the autumn of 2009. It concerned a female patient and a female member of my staff. I do not know whether them both being female has any bearing on the subject or not but I suspect it has.

I was a little busy that day so I asked the female member of staff to enter the cubicle where the patient was lying face up and to question the patient as to her condition. This is standard practice as it allows my staff to gain valuable practice in the art of questioning and the processing of the information gained by it. It also allows the patient to have a free reign and say anything without me being present. The latter is occasionally a very good thing because the mere presence of the practitioner may result in an unconscious tendancy by the patient to give a better than is state of their condition. I usually walk in at an appropriate moment and the member of staff normally gives me an ordered and succinct account..

As soon as I walked in I was immediately assailed by the overwhelming impression that there was not one, but two patients in the cubicle with me. Sure enough this was confirmed when the member of staff began to report on the patients condition. Instead of an orderly, reasoned account, it was ragged and incoherent with bits of information added almost as afterthought. In short it was something that I like to refer to as "a dogs dinner". It was the work of a sick person. An account of a diseased person recounted by the diseased. The member of staff had lost the POG and crossed over from empathy into total identification with the patient.

I smiled as I began to treat both of them.

1.2   THIS AND THAT

Everybody whether they like it or not, consciously or unconsciously seeks identification with something or someone. After some time, after some exposure, after some reflection, one realises that all of this is false and that the true being uses no such device, no crutch to arrive at the true.

Studying Oriental medicine can be an interesting path to tread because one hits, or is forced to examine, a number of obstacles along the way. The first that a Westerner or even a modern East Asian invariably comes up against is the difference in the way of thinking. This gap can be approached from a cultural view point where the "target culture" (in this case China, Korea, Japan, etc.) is "learned". In my experience this works in the initial period but in the end is doomed to failure. The following account, a true one, illustrates this.

I had been in Japan for a couple of years and made a brief trip to Sri Lanka. During my time in Japan, I tried to absorb as much as I could. This meant in my case and I suspect, in many others as well, a process by which I ate, slept and lived as close as I could to a Japanese lifestyle. In youthful folly, this meant that of course I avoided like the plague anything that was foreign. Food was Japanese—there was no problem there of course. Sleeping on my futon was beautiful. Japanese toilets were great exercise. Shoes—wooden geta (the one pronged type) proved to be a little bit noisy walking along the tarmac roads of my neighbourhood. The biggest anomaly though was that I actually found myself avoiding even eye contact with any foreigners for fear of having to talk to them.

Anyway, as I boarded the plane leaving Narita, I reflected that I had learned culturally and was therefore somehow a better person for it. Learning, real learning, never occurs within the constraints that we seek to impose on it.

On my second day in Sri Lanka, I sat down to lunch. An ordinary setting for an extraordinary event. I, eager to experience the local cuisine, ordered a traditional dish. Relishing in my new found cultural openness, I looked forward to the new culinary experience. When the dish arrived, my eyes rested on the contents of the meal for a while. To my dismay, I found that my tools of investigation merely consisted of two sets of bias. The rice was differently prepared from the Basmati that I was used to in England when eating Indian food. It was also different in colour and texture from the *Koshi Hikari* rice which I enjoyed so much in Japan. The taste was also different. But what was the taste? I couldn't even tell because I was in the grip of two sets of prejudices[2].

Now here I was after two years of considerable effort with the dubious luxury of having two of these sets. To make matters worse, the first set of prejudices I had unavoidably acquired but the second I had actually learned!

The fatal attraction to become lodged in preconceived ideas is not a recent development of the human race: the 81st chapter of the *Nan Ching* is a little nudge from the past to arise from the slumber.

第 八 十 一 難
八十一難曰. 經言. 無實實虛虛. 損 不足而益有
餘. 是寸口脉耶. 將病自有 虛實耶. 其損益奈
何. 然. 是病非謂寸口脉也. 謂病自有虛實 也.
假令肝實而肺虛. 肝者木也. 肺者 金也. 金木當
更相平. 當知金平木. 假 令肺實而肝虛微少氣.
用鍼不補其肝. 而反重實其肺. 故曰實實虛虛. 損
不足 而益有餘. 此者中工之所害也

---

[2] The type usually prevalent in the youth of any country, but a few extra special ones peculiar to the British.

81st Difficulty:

The eighty-first difficulty states that the classic[3] says that it is neither permissible to make excess more excess nor deficiency more deficient. Nor is it permissible to further diminish the lacking or to supplement the over abundant. Is this referring to the state of the inch opening pulse or is it the deficiency and excess of the disease itself? What is meant by 'further diminish' and 'supplement'?

The answer is as follows. This concerns the disease itself not the inch opening pulse. It is referring to the deficiency and excess of the disease itself. Let us take an example where the Liver is excess and the Lungs are deficient. The Liver is Wood and the Lungs are Metal. The Metal and Wood are of course in constant exchange to maintain a balance. It is of course known that Metal balances Wood. For example Lung Excess with Liver deficiency leads to minute Ki. If at this time acupuncture is performed not tonifying the Liver and conversely doubling the excess Lung, the excess becomes more excess and the deficient becomes more deficient. Diminishing the lacking and increasing the abundant; this is a common fault of the middle level practitioner.

The term "中工" which I have translated as middle level practitioner is translated as "mediocre" by Unschuld[4] I had long suspected myself of mediocrity, so have, I am sure, some of my patients. I decided to look into the *Nan Ching's* definition of mediocrity.

---

[3] This is referring to unknown medical classics embodying treatment methods that were prevalent at that time. They were obviously written a long time prior to the *Nan Ching* and sometimes appear to be a reference to the *Ling Shu* or the *Su Wen* but not always.

[4] "*Nan-Ching*: The Classic of Difficult Issues" Publ. Southern Materials Center, Inc., Taipei, 1986. Paul U. Unschuld.

The interesting thing about this last difficulty of the *Nan Ching* is that it asks us to think about the excess and deficiency of the disease itself. It expressly tells us to regard the disease and not the pulse. One might think that this is unusual in a book that seems to emphasise the pulse. It is fitting that the last difficulty should remind us not to focus on the pulse at the expense of diagnosis. Prejudiced ideas!

LEVELS OF PRACTITIONERS

The 13th chapter of the *Nan Ching* gives us more to consider:

十三難曰

...經言知一為下工，知二為中工，知三為上工。上工者十全九，中工者十全八，下工者十全六，此之謂也

13th Difficulty:

...The classic states knowledge of one results in a low level practitioner. Knowledge of two results in mediocre practitioner. Knowledge of three results in a high level practitioner. High level practitioners heal nine out of ten. Mediocre practitioners heal eight out of ten. Low level practitioners heal six out of ten. This is what is said here."

七十七難曰

七十七難曰．經言．上工治未病．中工治已病者何謂也．然所謂治未病者．見肝之病．則知肝當傳之與脾．故先實其脾氣．無令得受肝之邪．故曰治未病焉．中工治已病者．見肝之病．不曉相傳．但一心治肝．故曰治已病也

77th Difficulty:

The seventy-seventh difficulty states that the classic says the superior level practitioner heals the future disease, the

mediocre practitioner heals the present disease. What does this mean?

Actually the so called treatment of future disease is when finding Liver disease it is known that the Liver will surely transmit this to the Spleen as well. Therefore firstly make the Spleen Ki excess [stronger]. Doing this will not allow the Spleen to receive the Liver pathogen. This is called treating the future disease. The middle level [mediocre] practitioner treats the present disease and when finding Liver disease [the concept of] mutual transmission does not dawn on them. They single-mindedly treat only the Liver. This is called treating the present disease.

As we have seen, the lowest level of practitioner knows one type of diagnosis and manages to heal about 60 percent of patients. The practitioner will be making great effort but with still quite a low level of concentration. They will feel that they are doing their best. Often they will feel encouraged by this success rate and make excuses or rationalise their failures.

The middle level practitioner knows two methods of diagnosis and treats single-mindedly the disease that is present. Concentration is no problem at this level. This level of practitioner heals 80 percent of patients. For the normal person and the low level practitioner, this appears to be great success. However, as well as the change in clinical proficiency, there is also a change in outlook; this level of practitioner only remembers the 20 percent not cured.

The upper level of practitioner (I assume) knows all three types of diagnosis and heals 90 percent of patients. He or she has no concept of how many are healed, but only knows that incorporating the concept of treating the future disease (治未病) results in halving the failure rate of the mid level practitioner to 10 percent. Despite this clinical excellence, he or she appears to be less involved in the treatment than the lower levels of practitioner. This is because this practitioner has graduated from the equation "More Effort = Better Results" to the equation "Less (No) Effort = Better (Best) Results".

The sage chooses whether to treat the patient or not. The sage is not bound by normal human values. There is no equation to graduate from. His or her actions are like a force of nature that cannot be bought, sold or influenced. Of course there will be a 100 percent success rate because only those that can be cured will be treated.

TREATING THE FUTURE DISEASE (治未病)

This idea of treating a disease that is not yet present is not an idea unique to the *Nan Ching*; it is the key principle of the *Nei Ching*. In the *Ling Shu* chapter 55 it mentions the difference between the upper and lower level practitioners. The *Su Wen* chapter 2 uses the term "sage", or "holy man", "聖人" to describe one who does not even bother to treat the present disease but instead treats disease before it occurs. I guess when you reach the level of a sage, one loses the desire to interfere in the natural course of events. Oh yes, we must always remember that disease is always a part of nature. Prevention is not such a direct intervention and therefore can still harness nature's flexibility without much karmic baggage.

Clinically we can incorporate the concept of treating the future disease in ways including the following:

1. Treat the whole body.

By treating the whole body I mean that the body is looked at and treated as a unit; not in parts. So for instance if a patient comes in with a bad arm we should at least examine the shoulder and neck. Also it means that the physical, energetic and spiritual aspects are considered in treatment. So for instance, a patient may come in with tendonitis. When the neck and shoulders are examined they are also found to be really tight. Upon questioning, the patient has had a long history of stiff shoulders. The patient's pulse and abdomen reveal Spleen Deficiency with Liver Excess. Nothing even has to be said. You treat her for tendonitis but you also work on the underlying depression which may not have even fully manifested yet.

2. Use shallow needling

Many of you may prefer deeper needling but even in that case you should still include skin needling (*Hifu Shin*; 皮膚鍼) and shallower needling if possible. The skin can be used to tonify the *Ei Ki* (衛気), the defensive *Ki*. This means that the body will have a greater resistance to disease and therefore act as a preventative. Also when the skin is well conditioned, the opening and closing of the skin and the function of the Lung *Ki* is improved, which will prevent the first stages of Cold Damage (傷寒). This would effectively cut off the gateway to other diseases. The other reason for including shallower needling is that it involves much less pain. This means that patients will be more willing to come to you for various conditions. A common phenomenon with people that specialise in deeper needling is that they do not have such a variety of patients. The patient has to be in pain sufficient enough to over ride the pain involved when they receive treatment. This will not be the case for colds, Liver dysfunction, infertility, asthma, night terror in children, atopic eczema, etc.

So you will have less contact with the entire spectrum of disease and therefore less chance to treat people before they get really sick. I know of some practitioners who even ask their patients to cancel their appointments when they have a cold. This will not help them to prevent disease.

3. Treat the Gallbladder meridian

In most conditions, it is always worth checking out and treating the Gall Bladder meridian. This is because it will almost always be tender and reactive and classically speaking it is the "中正之宮[5]" which means that it balances the other organ meridian systems. The other reason is that it will prevent blood stagnation from building up. Blood stagnation is a big factor in serious disease and working on it is a big step in prevention.

4. Root Treatment

The root treatment can be used to treat disease that is present now but it is even more useful in treating for prevention (已病). Most problems can be treated by using the ideas contained in the *Su Wen* and the 69th chapter of the *Nan Ching*. These are namely the idea that all disease begins with a deficiency of one of the *Zang* organs and that this is often best treated by using the Mother-Child (constructive, 相生) relationship. Sometimes though, the controlling (相剋) relationship needs to be used to treat and prevent disease. The condition is often more serious than that where the constructive cycle is used.

CASE STUDY

History & Symptoms

A 42 year old man with a history of viral meningitis on a recurrent basis 4 or 5 times a year. He is a well trained athlete. Currently he suffers from insomnia, lack of energy, anxiety and lower back pain.

The abdomen shows a lack of resilience on the conception vessel below the navel and tightness of the epigastric region. There is heat in the chest.

Overall the pulse was fast and strong. The left proximal pulse was relatively sunken and wiry. The left medial pulse was strong and floating but deficient upon pressure. The right distal pulse was powerful and appeared to become more so upon pressure, i.e. a sunken pulse.

---

[5] This could be translated as the "Minister of Impartiality".

Treatment

He was basically Kidney deficient but due to his work commitments, he had become Liver *Yin* deficient. The heat that was normally radiated out was being trapped in the upper body causing the meningitis.

The needles were retained on the tight areas of the chest and abdomen. Two rounds of moxa, *Chi Netsu Kyu* (知熱灸)[6], were applied to *Dan Chu* (膻中; CV17) and one round each to the abdominal points. A root treatment consisting of tonification of *Fuku Ryu* (復溜; KI7), *Chu Ho* (中封; LV4), *Gyo Sai* (魚際; LU10) was performed. The patient was then turned face down, needles were retained on the upper back including the Governor Vessel and Needle Head moxibustion was performed on the left and right *Jin Yu* (腎俞; BL23) on the lower back. Moxa (*Chi Netsu Kyu*) was performed on the upper back at the end of the session. This treatment was repeated once a week for about 5 sessions and then he came in sporadically once a month or so. Over the course of two years he had viral meningitis only once or twice. He enjoyed a period of good health when basically his only symptoms were sports related lower back injuries. His treatment at that time often consisted of only a Kidney *Yin* Deficiency root treatment (tonification of KI7) and some deeper needling of the lower back and some lighter needling of the neck.

Then there was a gap of six months or so and the patient returned with meningitis at the time of treatment. He was so used to the symptoms by now that he did not need to go to the hospital. His symptoms were initially a loss of appetite (very unusual for him) followed by lethargy and a splitting headache. The symptoms and the pulse lead very easily to the diagnosis of Spleen Deficiency Liver Excess. Yes, I know you want me to tell you what the pulse was, so here goes. The pulse over all was fast, a little sunken and wiry with deficiency upon pressure at the right medial position and the left distal position. The left medial pulse was a

---

[6] See Articles 3.1 entitled "Introduction to Moxibustion" and Article 3.2 entitled "Clinical uses of Moxibustion" for an explanation of this technique.

little excess.

The epigastric area was tight and painful on pressure. The treatment consisted of tonification of *Dai Ryo* (大陵; PC7)) and *Tai Haku* (太白; SP3) followed by shunting of *Ashi Rin Kyu* (足臨泣; GB41).

The patient was then turned face down and touch needling was applied to the upper back and neck. The patient responded very well to the treatment, slept better that night and within 3 or 4 days was his old self again.

Observations

It became clear from observing the patient in the viral meningitis state that he was suffering from what would be called "*Shao Yang* disease" in the *Shang Han Lun*. This is often seen in patients that have a cold, take antibiotics, do not recover and then decide to visit their acupuncturist. It is best treated for Spleen Deficiency Liver Excess Heat syndrome.

My initial treatments were aimed at tonifying the *Yin* aspect of the Kidney and Liver and recirculating the heat stuck in the Lungs. This proved successful in treating his symptoms of anxiety, insomnia and lack of energy and clearing the heat that was stuck in his upper body. Basically the treatments returned him to his constitution (i.e. Kidney deficiency constitution) and that is why he enjoyed relatively good health. When he became sick with viral meningitis he exhibited Spleen Deficiency with Liver Excess Heat syndrome. This was a state which was out of his constitution and was therefore more serious. I knew how to treat this patient to keep in good health and heal his viral meningitis but I wanted to go one step further. So I pondered this for a while and on my teacher *Ikeda Sensei*'s suggestion I decided to move into treating the future disease or prevention by treating him for Spleen Deficiency whenever he came in.

This meant that I was preventing him from becoming Spleen Deficiency Liver Excess Heat syndrome which is the state that for him equals viral meningitis. At the same time I was also nudging his body into Kidney Deficiency by strengthening the Spleen which has a controlling action on the Kidneys. So even if this patient presents with Kidney deficiency pulse, I have been deliberately treating for Spleen Deficiency with good results thus far.

BALANCE OF POWER

Another application of treating the disease before it manifests is to think about the state of peace (health) as a state of balanced aggressive tension. Unfortunately there is very rarely peace, love and understanding. It is often peace gained through a balance of power(s). If the truth be known, *Yin* and *Yang* are not harmonious entities but rather two opposing forces. When one is weaker than the other, the stronger one becomes dominant and vice versa. This may not be the ideal state of affairs for man, but this is nature that has ideals beyond anything man can conceive of. In terms of the five phases, this means that each unit is most easily pressurised by the controlling phase. So for instance, Metal is said to control Wood.

Physiologically this means that the function of the Lung meridian to circulate *Ki* and radiate outwards will oppose the gathering action of the Liver meridian on the Blood. It is not actually the Metal cutting the Wood - but the threat of it that is energetic. If the Metal actually cuts the Wood, it is physical and it can only occur a finite number of times. This means you do not get much energetically for your money.

The archetypal energies of the five phases are energetically infinite. Thus the Lung *Ki* circulation has no desire of its own to hinder the Liver meridian, but its function - its very existence - causes it. A bit like a husband at a party with his wife; there is never any real freedom or sense of "party" for either of them. So in the root treatment we can add a point or two to ensure that the deficiency is not only tonified but there can be an energetic confidence to relax and continue to enjoy functioning properly. For example if there is a root treatment for Liver

Yang Deficiency, as well as tonifying *Tai Kei* (太谿; KI3) and *Tai* Sho (太衝; LV3), we can also tonify *Fuku Ryu* (KI7) and *Chu Ho* (LV4). Wood fears Metal most. These last two points represent the Metal points and are used to allay the fear of the Wood so that it can function freely and leisurely.

For Kidney Deficiency, *Tai Kei* (KI3) is added to protect from the Earth. For Spleen Deficiency, *In Paku* (隱白; SP1) is added to protect from the Wood. For Lung Deficiency, *Gyo Sai* (LU10) is added to protect from the Fire.

CONCLUSIONS

Learning can increase stupidity. Real learning makes you free. One prejudice is better than two.

We must be aware that when we begin our studies, we begin with a pure intention of doing our best. Then after some learning we get contaminated with techniques and theories. If after that, we get into real learning, we can begin to really care again.

The hand is the Heart in physical form. At the centre of the palm is the fire point (Heart) of the Pericardium (energetic *Yang* of the Heart) meridian. To treat from the Heart automatically means that the touch is true and the *Ki* flows well.

1.3 WHATS IN A NAME? MERIDIAN THERAPY, TJM & THE CLASSICS

FIRST IMPRESSIONS CAN BE DECEPTIVE

When I first encountered meridian therapy (or *Keiraku Chiryo* (経絡治療), as it is known in Japanese), I decided on the spot that I never wanted to practise this style of acupuncture or be associated with any of its practitioners. It seemed to me at that time that most practitioners were individuals who had failed at the other things they had attempted during their lives. Whenever they gathered together, these past failures gave an air of despair to the occasion. After several hours of study with these practitioners I would have to revive myself with a strong coffee and a sandwich at one of the ubiquitous nearby Japanese coffee shops. While sipping the steaming, percolated black liquid, I would feel my body revive and the suicidal gloom evaporate.

At that time I also met some Chinese-style TCM acupuncturists. The atmosphere of their meetings was completely different: they were always willing and able to argue problems theoretically, and the study groups were in general animated affairs with a feeling of solidity.

These general feelings can be summarized using a real-life example. At a social occasion, I met two gentlemen, one Chinese, the other Japanese. After exchanging niceties with the Chinese gentleman, I asked him what he did for a living. He looked me straight in the eye and with pride replied that he was an acupuncturist. When I put the same question to the Japanese gentleman, the content of the answer was the same, but the form of the reply differed remarkably. He became seemingly nervous and disorientated for a moment before mumbling under his breath that he too was an acupuncturist. Further enquiry revealed that he was a practitioner of meridian therapy.

Having said all this, why would anyone want to practise meridian therapy? The answer has to be no one unless they are seriously considering suicide. However, please read on and I will try to demonstrate why meridian therapy is worthy of being practised.

The turning point was the first treatment I received from *Masakazu Ikeda Sensei*, probably the leading light of meridian therapy and now my teacher. Previous to this, I had made it a policy to try out people who had a good reputation as practitioners. However, until my meeting with *Ikeda Sensei*, the only person that had inspired me to study with them was *Misao Takenouchi Sensei*. There was no question that *Ikeda Sensei* could talk a great fight: his books and lectures are superb. The question was, could he perform clinically? I had tried virtually all the "big" names, so in some ways I was the joker in the pack as I lay down ready to receive a treatment and find out whether *Ikeda Sensei* could match words with actions. He proved his worth immediately: I felt *Ki* literally bubbling out of *Ikeda Sensei*'s hands and down the needles, sizzling its way through my meridians. All this with the needle only inserted about 1 mm, meaning that I was experiencing regulation of *Ki* in its purest form. The beautiful technique, combined with *Ikeda Sensei's* wisdom and humour, was awe inspiring. In short, this was the type of treatment that I wanted to give my patients and this was the type of person I wanted to become. Thus I unconsciously chose to learn how to be a good oriental medical practitioner, not how to practise good oriental medicine.

This choice is important for a number of reasons. First, it allows knowledge to be absorbed via the solid matrix of the teacher and his approach to life, which includes qualities such as wisdom, generosity, humour, and patience, all of which allow knowledge to be used properly. Second, it allows the intangibles that lubricate or animate all the more obvious qualities to be absorbed in a natural way, often without the teacher or student being aware. Third, it allows us the great joy and benefit of a relationship with the teacher, of caring for him or her in a real, personal way and being cared for in return. This represents a legacy of learning of such great proportions that it will never die and will always be of value, irrespective of the millennium. This is the traditional method.

WHAT'S IN A NAME?

The name "meridian therapy," which I do not particularly like, may infer that other styles of acupuncture do not use meridians. Of course, this is not true. At the time of meridian therapy's inception, Japanese acupuncture had been streamlined (some would say castrated) by a government anxious to raise the standard of western medicine and to outlaw the inefficient folk medicine of the time. The result was that acupuncture consisted of a list of points and the disease types for which they were to be used. Treatment often consisted solely of inserting needles where the patient told the practitioner to do so. Thus acupuncture at this time was completely point based, with no thought being given to regulating the meridians to cure disease. It was in this situation that the term "meridian therapy" was coined to distinguish this style of practice, almost in a reactionary way, from the style prevalent at the time. Therefore in terms of usage, the term "meridian therapy" has a history similar in duration to TCM.

I have always preferred to use the term "classical acupuncture" instead of meridian therapy because the style is based on the classics. "Classics" itself is a slightly nebulous term, but for these purposes there are five: the *So Mon* (素問; Simple Questions); *Rei Su* (霊枢; Spiritual Pivot); *Nan Gyo* (難経; Classic of Difficult Issues); *Sho Kan Ron* (傷寒論; Classic of Cold Diseases); and the *Kin Ki Yo Ryaku* (金匱要略; Prescriptions from the Golden Chest).

One thing to bear in mind is that classical acupuncture is not the only style of acupuncture used in Japan and is by no means the most popular, being used by a minority of practitioners; the situation is unlikely to change for some time. The only reason that I am currently practising classical acupuncture is that it is the most effective style I have encountered—effective in that it is clinically superb and that it is a vehicle that allows development of the practitioner. The range of skills and information that has to be assimilated demands much physical and mental effort. This aspect makes one's studies spill over into all aspects of one's being and life, ensuring its popularity among those who are willing to persevere on the one hand and its minority status on the other. For some people it may seem like too much work for too little reward.

On a recent lecture tour, *Ikeda Sensei* coined the term TJM (Traditional Japanese Medicine) to describe classical acupuncture. This term is appropriate, for a number of reasons. First, it distinguishes this style from other Japanese styles which are not traditional. This is important because there is still a tendency to put all the varied styles together and label them the "Japanese approach," which is a mistake. Second, it shows that its most recent origin (its ancient origin is China) is Japan. Third, it includes by definition not just acupuncture but also moxibustion, *Do In* (導引) massage, *Ki* strengthening exercises, blood letting, dietetics, and herbs. The need for this new name is similar to that which existed when the term meridian therapy was coined. At that time, a name was needed to distinguish the style from other practises within Japan. Now, it is necessary to distinguish between TJM and TCM, which is practised worldwide. However, I hope that in future there will be less need to label acupuncture styles, with all the sometimes unfortunate connotations these labels have in people's minds. Until then, TJM is the preferred term.

CHARACTERIZING TJM—SINISTER TENDENCIES?

I am like most acupuncturists: I love to needle. And not just shallow needling, which is what some people assume TJM is about, but also deep, strong needling. However, the first comment that people often make when they see TJM for the first time is that the needling is light and shallow. They go on to say that it cannot be effective and must be a special Japanese invention necessary for their delicate constitution or culture.

But TJM involves much more than shallow needling. For instance, there are the various implements involved: the *Shin Kan* (鍼管; needle tube), the *Tei Shin* (錠鍼; a type of thick blunt needle[7]), the "shark's fin" (one of my favourites), and other tools that I experiment with in the clinic, as well as needles of all lengths and sizes. As mentioned above, TJM also incorporates moxibustion, *Do In* massage (導引), *Ki* strengthening exercises, blood letting, dietetics, and herbs.

Perhaps the most defining characteristic of the TJM that I practise is the extensive use of the left hand to press, knead, stroke, pinch, and tap, and use of the mind to bring the *Ki* to the various areas. This sinister aspect also surprises many first-time observers of TJM; the use of the left hand to massage, probe, and sense *Ki* appears mysterious and unfathomable to some, who think that this again must be a Japanese invention. This view is particularly prevalent among college and university students who are actively encouraged to use pincers and in some cases gloves, thereby treating patients without ever touching them in some cases! However, the importance of the left hand and light (and heavy) needling have been known for a long time.

Of all the classics, the *Nan Ching* (難経; Classic of Difficulties) is one of the most popular, innovative, and refined concerning acupuncture. Three chapters from this text (chapters 71, 78, and 80), amongst others, support the use of the left hand and also illustrate my point that TJM is based firmly on the classics.

The Chinese text of chapter 71 of the *Nan Ching* reads (words in brackets in my translation are my additions):

難曰：經言刺榮無傷衛，刺衛無傷榮，何謂也

In the sacred text it mentions that when needling the nutritive [Ki], the defensive [Ki] must not be damaged. Conversely,

---

[7] See Article 2.1 entitled "The Needling Truth"

when needling the defensive [Ki] one must not damage the nutritive [Ki]. What does this mean?

然：鍼陽者，臥鍼而刺之；刺陰者，先以左手攝按所鍼榮俞之處，氣散乃內鍼。是謂刺榮無傷衛，刺衛無傷榮也。

When needling the Yang [defensive Ki], the needles should be inserted so that they lie flat; when needling the Yin [nutritional Ki], the left hand should first be used to press and knead the area, clearing it of defensive [Ki]. The point formed by this process should then be needled. In this way, when needling the nutritive [Ki], the defensive [Ki] is not damaged and vice versa.

This chapter hints at a style of light needling for defensive *Ki* and massage to an area before deeper insertion when aiming at the nutritive *Ki*. This in turn indicates that needling should be painless and treatment touch oriented. Light needling in particular is essential for a *Yang*-deficient patient because heavier needling will lead to a worsening of the condition. Furthermore, if deeper needling is necessary, pressing and kneading alert the patient to the fact that this type of needling is needed and prepare the tissues, revealing the point.

In Chinese, chapter 78 of the *Nan Ching* reads (words in brackets in my translation are my additions):

難曰：針有補瀉，何謂也

What is meant by tonification and dispersion using needles?

然：補瀉之法，非必呼吸出內針也。然：知為鍼者，信其左；不知為針者，信其右。當刺之時，必先以左手厭按所

It is not [absolutely] necessary to needle according to the

> *breathing cycle. Knowledgeable practitioners actually put faith in their left hands. Practitioners who do not know put faith in their right hands. Before insertion it is important first to press and knead the area...*

This chapter deals with the methods of tonification and dispersion, which are (or should be) the cornerstone of treatment, and is emphatic regarding the emphasis that should be placed on the left hand. This chapter also automatically implies a style of treatment emphasizing touch, sensitivity, and the ability to feel and regulate *Ki*. At the other end of the spectrum is the practitioner who relies mainly on the right hand. This implies a style in which there is less emphasis on touch and the primary objective is to get the needles in. I refer to this style of needling as "plonking," but the *Nan Ching* is not as kind and refers to it as the work of those who "do not know."

The final chapter I would like to consider is chapter 80 (words in brackets in my translation are my additions):

> 難曰：經言有見如入，有見如出者，何謂也
>
> *The sacred text says when it is seen, enter, and when it is seen, leave. What does this mean?*
>
> 然：所謂有見如入者，謂左手見氣來至，乃內針；針入見氣盡，乃出針。是謂有見如入，有見如出也。
>
> *'When it is seen' refers to the arrival of Ki as seen [or felt] by the left hand, at which time the needle should be inserted. [In the other case,] 'when it is seen' refers to when Ki is felt to be at it's fullest, when the needle should be extracted. This is what is meant by 'when it is seen, enter, and when it is seen, leave'.*

This chapter again refers to the left hand being used to monitor the state of the patient's *Ki* to determine the amount of stimulation suitable.

These extracts from the *Nan Ching* illustrate that TJM stresses ancient Chinese practices, and these are currently enjoying a renaissance in Japan. However, everyone can benefit from this, irrespective of race, colour, creed, or label. These practices, carefully preserved and handed down through the ages, are now available to those willing to invest the time, effort, and energy necessary to train diligently. Now that you have an idea of the roots of TJM, you can decide wisely how you want to practise.

1.4 CLINIC CONVERSATIONS

The following are extracts of actual conversations in the clinic between the author and his *"understandents"*[8]. They cover a range of different topics, were recorded at different times and involve different people (as indicated). This section is therfore intended to be read as individual snippets or glimpses rather than to flow as the development of a single idea or theme.

ACCEPTANCE / NON-ACCEPTANCE BY THE PATIENT

EO: With the root treatment the mechanics are only there to get you in place. Once you are there, then you need to be relaxed and then.... Big....Full. You are not stopping at the hands. They are just access points and now you go into the patient. And beyond her.

We have to forget at this time the techniques and everything else. Otherwise you get stuck at the hands. It's like a *tsubo*[9]. You can get stuck there, but it is a way of accessing the meridian. Of course if you get the point spot on then you get better access. But you have to use it just as the tool that it really is. You see, in many cases you get people going on about the *oshide*[10]. Of course it will change depending on where I want to treat. So the mechanics – yes – there is a period where you concentrate on the mechanics. But we still have to put that in it's place. It is just mechanics. It is not the be-all and end-all. You need the mechanics in place so that you can utilize the *Ki*.

So when you have found what you believe to be the point, your hands are there anyway. Give your left hand to the patient. You can have the right hand if you want. Connect them up and blow *Ki* into them. Fill

---

[8] A term coined by the author to describe a practitoner whose efforts are focused toward **understanding** through learning and practise of the art. The distinction with the term "student" is explored in an Article entitled "Not The Sharpest Knife In The Draw - Speculations On Learning" in Vol III of *A Long Road.*
[9] An acupuncture point.
[10] 押し手 – This character is literally translated as the "the pushing/ holding hand".   In refers to the position/ shape of the non-needling hand (usually the left).

them up. Don't worry – it's not your *Ki*. You are not living in isolation from the universe. The more you realise that the better. Then at the end of the treatment the patient should feel a little bit happier – a little bit less lonely – a little bit more included.

TS: But this is why the attitude of the patient is important – if they are not willing to accept it then they won't feel that.

EO: Well – if we bring up the idea of acceptance then immediately when you bring up this idea, it means that we are not accepting their non-acceptance. In the beginning I would try to work on that. But now I realise you just have to let them have it. It is a bit like a weight sitting in the way. You can try to move it. But if you slowly fill that place up with water (or *Ki*) then it begins to move anyway. We fill them up so much that their non-acceptance eventually is ineffective.

We can talk them down. Yes, but then our mind is full of their non-acceptance. It becomes the issue of contention. So you have to be a little bit careful. I have tried both ways, but I prefer the latter. Of course it depends on the case. You can try both ways and then come back to me in a couple of years to tell me I am right.

TEMPERANCE

EO: This applies to you, TS. I like your enthusiasm. You want to do it all – and you want to do it now – to bring about change. I know this because I used to be the same. It's good. But in my experience, this will lead in one of 2 directions. Either to disillusionment - as the world will not react and change in the way you want it to. Or otherwise to Temperance – where you understand more about the process of change. You need to understand where the person is and what is possible. Let's take that last patient as an example. You can come in hard and fast and make demands but she will feel guilty and avoid you and won't come back. Then we don't even get the chance. Or, we take the slow approach – water dripping over time – this way she comes back and we have the chance to allow change to evolve of itself –

NON-INTERFERENCE

(In discussing a patient case and whether he should be spoken to about his approach and condition)

EO: Now you see – the other bigger picture is that we are here to gain some experiences here in this life. We could live in a little bubble – and eat apple pie – and watch the Johnny Carson show – and be happy, and never want or need nothin'. But we won't get much of an experience.

So we have to experience various things. We have to go through it. I don't want to interfere with that. I will help people, but I am getting a bit clearer about the idea of non-interference.

When I was doing *Kan Yu* (肝俞；BL17) on AY – I felt the effect of her parents there. I had no desire to feel that. Don't connect this with sense or anything. I was just neutral.

TS: When you say this... ...where in you is forming this realization...is it a sensation?

EO: It's like an encoded signal. I don't create it. You could think of it like a zip file that comes in and then you expand it. For me there is no doubt – it is absolutely real. I want to be very clear about it. Because you see some people who go off into imaginary areas – it's all very pleasant and all that... But I don't invite it or think about it or look for it. Otherwise there is a chance that my prejudices and conditioned experience can affect what I feel. Even when I do that there is still a possibility that it is still going on.

But of course – I know that I am better than I was let's say 10 years ago. But here's the interesting thing. In the beginning the experience was an accumulative process that allowed me to improve. But recently I would say that the experience that is increasing is allowing me to let go of more – and allow me to improve. So it's important to understand this process which I presume we all go through. I spoke about this before – in terms of deconstructing myself. You see, at that time I wanted to do better than myself and I could see that myself was the limiting factor. So I knew that I had to change somehow.

So there is no particular charm or fascination with it. If it comes it comes. If it doesn't - like in the case of that young fella we just treated – then it doesn't. You see in some places they are looking for this element each time – looking for this psycho-emotional component. And actually they do it a dis-service because it is already there – it doesn't need to be looked for. If you are looking, you are involving striving – then there will always be a restraint on the *Ki* – it won't be free-flowing.

WHAT DOES THIS PERSON ACTUALLY NEED?

EO: Getting them better as quickly as possible is just *one* of the factors here. For instance sometimes I could get people better quicker but it might be too much for their work schedule or whatever. So you have to take various factors in. One of the factors is to consider 'what does this person actually need at this time?'. Do they really need to have every ailment dealt with? Or are theit ailments actually an indicator telling them that, yes, they *are* drinking too much – or they *are* not sleeping enough – or they *are* overeating. Of course, we can take the edge off it – and sometimes of course we can take the whole symptom away – but this will be more or less useless in the long term. It is far better if we take the edge off the symptoms and bring them to an understanding of where they are now.

We see these processes many times. They don't – all they see is their own process.

HEALTH

Patient: How can this fix my knee? I have osteo-arthritis.

EO: Well – it depends what you are looking for. You may think you are looking for a cure to osteo-arthritis. But the truth is you are looking for a cure to your pain – and freedom from your perceived inability to use your body as you wish. So – we look at the energetic function and underpinning to all the structures – the muscle, tendon, fascia, bone, blood-flow, nerve activity – and we work on *how* they are working. Our view is not about having perfect structure- you can have perfect structure and be dead... ...We are more interested in the energetic functioning. So perhaps your bone will not re-generate to the perfect state – but if you are pain-free and have the use of your body, does this really matter?

IS IT MAKING YOU HEALTHY?

EO: Yes, I agree "eating vegetables is healthier than meat" I agree with that 100%, but why are we doing it? If we say we are doing it for moral reasons, then OK we have that in mind, and then the health is second. That's OK and you are clear about it. But, if you are someone in this particular profession and you say you are eating it for your health, and it isn't leading to good health, then we have to look again. It's the same as when patients tell me they are eating a certain health food... I ask them a simple question, "Is that diet making you healthy?" and if the answer is "No", then don't call it a health food diet. You have seen this yourself right. This is a matter not just for you, AY, but for all of us. Every day, I try to take away more and more bullshit until I can see a little bit more clearly. It never ends.

A NICE CUP OF TEA

EO: When I make a cup of tea it is rounded – I could show you how I do it but then all you will have is a solution to that problem. I want you to work out how to find that solution – how to generate it – in any situation. Then you can apply our learning to everything. Through the tea you make I can see the mentality behind it.

You don't make it by putting it on and leaving it – you decide that you are going to do it – and you stay with it. In the same way I put the needles in number 3 bed and then I leave the cubicle, I am still there – connected to what is going on. I don't put it down, no matter what else I am doing – then it comes to me when it is the right time for the next step.

It's the same in life – no matter what you are doing, you are still connected in some small way at least, to all the things which influence you.

HELP

EO: What I see with a lot of people is that they cheat themselves out of a chance to learn. People can spend years and years getting better at cheating themselves. Does this ring home? I mean you can only going to come along this path once – and you are given the chance to learn and change – So when there is the chance, we might as well try to respond to it at least. Usually the compromises and excuses are ways of cheating yourself out of ways to grow. So respond. Take the chance.

SR: Actually my condition today is not so good. I think I need your help.

EO: I am helping you – that's exactly what I am doing. Like for instance – I helped you when you were about to set fire to your clothes today. That's the best help. I could have been really kind and not said anything – and then you would be on fire. You see you need to be careful about what "help" means for you. What you really mean by help is that you want me to understand you. I already do – I know that. I know where you are coming from I was there – I am in there too. But the truth is that most people don't really want to be understood - they just want what they want. You know – if you can't see what's really wrong then sometimes it's better not to help. You can be kind – but that's not the same.

SETTING YOURSELF UP FOR FAILURE

EO: So after being here now for a certain length of time it is more difficult to comprehend what people imagine acupuncture should be – or to imagine the way to learn it. There are a number of mechanisms going on. One is that people want to set themselves up for failure. Because it is much easier to have a teacher that is oriental and to believe that he is good *because* he is oriental…or 5th generation or whatever… And the other is that people are always looking for heroes – then they can let go of the responsibility of improving themselves. Another is that they want to present it as some sort of cultural thing. Yes, we can say that it came out of China. But what they are talking about is actually about universal principles. Not even just human principles. Not even just natural principles…. Actually *universal* principles. That's how great what they left us is. And it should be looked at in that light. If you always approach it as some kind of cultural delicacy then you will never get to grips with it.

This cultural discrepancy is not really it. Because if you are learning something that is genuine, not only are you learning something that is beyond your technical ability. It is also actually beyond your realm of cognition. Your realm of actual experience. This is the same for a Japanese, Chinese, Korean, English…you just have to be open and come in and try to learn. And having seen people of all races trying to learn it – and myself too, and seeing many people – it's not about culture really. Obviously if you know the Chinese characters and what have you, you have an advantage. But there are really good people who don't know them. We already have our own limitations – we really don't need to add to them… Anyway, just go for it.

AN UN-FURROWED BROW

TS: I can't understand – with that patient…

EO: Ok – stop there. What makes you think you can understand her. And also, you haven't got any… …duty to understand. It's alright. So let go of that. Now talk. You see – you feel better already….

TS: Well – when she comes in – she seems light enough – she chats with the other patients – and you let her do it – she seems ok. But as soon as she comes through and is involved in herself…

EO: Yes – we are investigating it. But look – what happens if we look at it with a non-furrowed brow. No- seriously – because it changes our method of investigation. Also the subject. We can affect the subject in this way. So now we have even changed the subject. The thing that we are investigating will change. Especially when we are dealing with humans – depending on the attitude we take. So, we are going to investigate bit by bit.

PROCEEDING & STOPPING

TS: Ah – ok – now I can feel something here…

EO: Yes. The reason being that you weren't out to push it from here or feel it from here or whatever…you just went out to feel. You can only feel what is there, right? But if you go out to specifically feel with the left or with the right in a certain way, then you are not really feeling what is there – you are conditioning it. You condition what you are trying to feel and then it's not feeling. It's just another form of conditioning. You just feel it and go in. Just go out to feel. Just press neutrally. And if it's not there, then go somewhere else.

I am scraping the bone now… this is what I'm after. If I really want to clear it then I want to scrape like this. But this is nothing really….it's child's play. Any mug can do this. It's not worth putting too much time into.

TS: So where should we be putting the time then?

EO: Into proceeding.

TS: A suitably enigmatic response....

EO: When you are not proceeding, you are stopping. When you are stopping, that's it – finished. And stopping can have various reasons. Stopping because you don't know the way. Or, and this is actually more common, stopping because you *think* you know the way. When you think you know it, you have stopped – that's it. Good night...

TS: What about when you *know* that you don't know it.

EO: Then.... ... you haven't even proceeded.

TS: How long should I leave these needles in then *Sensei*?

EO: Leave them in till next week... ...anyway, you are getting there, TS. Don't make the small mistakes – get those out of the way and you will be much better...

MIND AND SENSITIVITY.

EO: You have to balance the two. Try and use the mind where it is needed. If you have any doubts as to when not to use it, just watch these two. They always use it at the wrong time. Just do the opposite and you will be ok.

As far as the sensitivity is concerned, let that come out gradually. I don't want you to use the sensitivity. The way that you use it is you let it come out. You don't use it. You let it use you. But with the mind, you use it. You don't let it use you. This is the big difference between sensitivity – or shall we say the sub-conscious, and the conscious. Or the analytical and the intuitive. One you use very clearly. You don't let it occupy you.

You occupy it. You decide what you want done. There is a clear objective. The other one – you let it come out.

WU WEI

EO: OK, I'm a little more experienced than you. The other thing is, I'm not as attached to the outcome as you are. So, if they get better, of course I'm happy, but if they don't, I know that I'm doing my best for them. Remember, a lot of these people have had a hard time with western medicine as well... ...Anyway, I'm prepared to stay with them if they come in. And to help them along. But sometimes I can't do it in a short time.

So, that gives me a breathing space and allows me to give them a better quality of treatment. This idea of not being attached to the outcome is actually a very philosophical one that is expressed as *Wu Wei* (無為). This is not profound, no it's about daily blood and guts when you're trying your best. When you're not attached to the outcome, you see things much more clearly. So for example, say the patient comes in and I want to get as much money out of him as possible. If I'm attached to that, then I will end up talking a little strangely and he will pick up on it. If, on the other hand, I come in and say, I'm making enough money already...and think, "he can give me money or not I don't care"... what happens?

GW: He`s more at ease..

EO: Also, I look at him as a human being. With you now the issue of his neck is in the front of your mind, so basically - you're not seeing him. He is already panicky about his neck and then you add to it by just thinking about his neck....? Now, on a very facile level, it looks like you care about him, but it's not actually extending as far as him,... it's only about one portion of his neck. So, when that comes in, then we lose the *Wu Wei*.

Whereas, if I go to him and say "that's terrible. OK, let's see what we can do".... then things begin to open up again.

Don't be so concerned about the outcome.. I tell you why. The mere fact that you have opened a clinic and are wearing this white coat ...it means that you have already made the initial investment of wanting to help them.. It's already there. You don't want to add to it. If anything, you want to take away from it so that you can treat in a more enlightened and more illuminating way... you are free.

Do you see what I'm saying.. this is something that we all learn over time and something that we hear about... and people will use it in a nice beautiful way, without giving you the place that it came from... it came from real blood and guts.

Despite the meaning of the characters 無為 individually, it doesn't mean that you don't do anything. Rather, it's actually a very efficient way of using your energy. Another one is 行為 which is action, the opposite.

SYMPTOMS

EO: "Symptom free"...this does not define health. Health is more like the ability to deal with stuff – we are dynamic and live in a dynamic universe – like a tracker fund – moving as an approximation. Otherwise we are dead – that may be structurally perfect but with no life. For example – many macrobiotic people – they may be symptom free but in many cases they are like this simply because they are so weak they do not have enough energy to mount a defence (phlegm/ a cold is a sign of a body in defensive mode).

So there are a lot of symptoms but mostly the process is the same in a lot of cases. The needle is not the medicine – the medicine is the self-adjustment mechanism – but people lose touch with that through stress etc. Treatment can help people to re-learm this ability – so can meditation.

A COSMIC CRIME

EO: I don't want to waste my time. This is important. When you come in here you have to decide. If it's really really tight – then ok – you can spend some time here. For this person. But for another person you can go there and it can be over in 10 seconds. There is no standard time. You spend a lot of time here and often when I come and look at it, I realise it wasn't worth it. That means – and I'm serious – space time and energy has been misused. It's a bit like you have a magnifying glass and you want to concentrate on certain areas. If you look at the whole thing all you get is a lot of nothing. No – take a good look and then you come in like this on the places where it is needed. It is like a crime. A cosmic crime. I want you to move with all of this. And then when something needs attention, naturally it will go. When she calls me, I answer. When I call SR, she's out in the kitchen[11]... this is the natural order. When you come this way, I go that way... ...it's like a dance. Otherwise it's just a set of procedures. And that will only help a certain percentage. It won't actually have a life of its own. Even computers – they say, in another 15 years, are going to have a consciousness. And this, what we are doing, this is between *humans!*

INFORMATION & INSPIRATION

EO talks about a current project to translate *Ikeda Sensei's Nan Gyo Shin Gi* into English.[12]

You have to have a certain level to understand the depth of the commentary. It's a very good commentary. But you see - You can be impressed by the principle and the mind behind it which has got it. This will stimulate you to go on and investigate it yourself. *Or...* you can

---

[11] SR is an assisting practitioner who has the remarkable capacity to be always exactly not where she is needed. She manages to combine this with a unique ability to do the opposite of what is asked of her.

[12] An in-depth translation and commentary (in Japanese) on the *Nan Jing* (Classic of Difficult Issues) called 難経真義 (*Nan Gyo Shin Gi*; roughly meaning "*Nan Jing*: The True Meaning").

read the commentary as information. Reading it as information – maybe a lot of people do it – but for me it's a little bit of a waste. Because the most important thing about *Ikeda Sensei* is the inspiration. And that you go away not just with the information but also with an idea that "oh – I need to study this a little bit more.." and "oh – I haven't looked at that...". So you need to change the way you look at it. We are so brainwashed into looking at things in terms of information. In terms of hard currency. But actually more important is the principle – or the energetics behind it. *Then* you can use it for anything.

TAI CHI AS INVESTIGATION

EO: OK One of the things I often say about the *Tai Chi* practice is, basically, it's just another investigation. I go here, then I go there.. I put my hand up, Oh then it comes down... I put my weight back, Oh, it goes forward... I turn this way, Oh, I turn that way. It's based on absolutely sound, profound logic. There's no other word for it.. and it's investigating the way we move.. You see, the way that we move when we are relaxed which is slowly, smoothly... it's just using the mechanism that's all out there. So, actually, you are investigating the mechanism out there through that... that's what I feel recently. And they say that you practice in the beginning, you learn the order of things etc.. the mind is occupied (I put my leg here, I feel tight here, whatever). Then it says that you get to a stage where you more you practice, the more you develop. It makes a point of saying that it doesn't occur in the beginning. Why? I think it means that then you're not worried about whether your hands are here or whatever... but that you are just investigating the principle.

It's the same with acupuncture.. when I first started I was thinking "Oh this point is 3 units from xxx etc, I have to pay the rent etc" ..and then I got really tired, and when I got tired I just put a few needles in and they got better. I didn't know why. Probably at that time, I was so tired, not by design, I actually went with the principle because I had nothing left.. I didn't have any resistance. So, bit by bit I was able to apply that kind of principle when not being tired.

TS: This is the same as learning a language when once you get to a certain stage you accelerate more.

EO: Yes, but when we say that the development is quicker etc.. this is all a very comforting world to be in... ...but, quicker relative to what? You see, when we talk about things in terms of relativity, then it means that the investigation is beginning to grind to a halt. Because still we are relating it to what happened before. And when I relate, it means that that part of me which is relating isn't actually in investigation. It isn't actually open. It's OK to do that every now and again as just a little check, but as far as the basic principle, you have to even let go of that. Even that has to go. They say that normal learning, you add more and more. When you practice the Way or whatever you want to call it, then it's less and less. Even the idea of giving up, you have to give it up.

KATAS AND KOANS

EO: In this *Kata* the practice was one where they would go very tight but it's combined with the breath. So, that's where you have absolute tension.

GW: That's another rebound-effect?

EO: Yes, the more you are able to tighten, the more you will be able to relax afterwards. It's like a thing called static contraction.

TS: So, are you saying that following that theory, I should tighten my mind up more to then relax it more after...? *(in jest)*

EO: This is similar to when they give someone a *Koan*. A riddle that has no answer. So, the person goes to work with the only tool that he knows which is his conscious mind, but it is just like a problem that cannot be solved or a weight that can't be moved.. you contract and contract and contract and your mind searches and searches for the answer until it is totally exhausted and has exhausted all possibilities… then what is left after that? They sometimes call it `no mind` but it's not actually nothing, it's more everything than nothing.

TS: The problem with the *Koan*s I have read is that I look at it and realise that it's the same problem that I have with Christianity: OK I know that this has no answer so there's no point in using my mind to try and go into it.

EO: Now, I'll give you something that may help you. The trouble is that you are not emotionally involved in it. In that *Koan*, for example. That's why you have a teacher and a teacher gets you emotionally involved so that you know - from your own experience - that you just can't do it… Like the standing… I wouldn't have done it if Jan Diepersloot or *Sifu* weren't around to show it to me. I mean, why would I want to just stand around?! When you are in that situation and you have decided to study with a teacher, you have decided that what you have seen in the world isn't for you and you want to get to the heart of things.. …then you become emotionally involved and that's when humans can actually use what people normally think have to be suppressed all the time. We utilize this *(motions to his body/ heart)* again. It's like they talk of the five emotions.. people think to be healthy they have to be suppressed,

No they have to be in balance. It's the emotional content that gets us involved – it's what allows us to go a little bit further and really, if you like, break the mould.

TS: So, with the *Koan* there is a Buddhist master who sets a *Koan* for his student…

EO: Yes - But it's not a *Koan* that was for you that you have been reading. He is not your master and it wasn't set for you so there is no emotional involvement. That's the difference.

TS: Yes, then is that master then expecting that student to come back …. How does the student demonstrate that he has gone through the process of thinking about it? He could just come back and just say, "I've understood it"

EO: Then the master would beat him severely. Or perhaps just say, "OK you have learnt all you can from me… goodbye." No No No… you can see it in the way people move, the way they act. I'm not one of those masters, so I can't speak for them. But it's not about coming back with a clever answer. It's about making a fundamental change in themselves. That's the whole purpose of it So, they could speak eloquently about the answer but if there hasn't been a change, then there's nothing.

LEARNING OR BUYING A PRODUCT?

EO: What is best is that you have a look and decide what you want. I want you to be careful about being taught and about being sold something. These are 2 completely different things. A lot of people misinterpret the end product as all being the same.

Take DN - one of my students – he wanted to give people the chance to study the real thing. But now he understands that people to some extent also get what they are looking for. So when people want to go in and get a little bit of this – a little bit of that – it's a bit like shopping. And they pay for a product and that is what they get.

Actually *learning* the art is completely different. In the end – if you want to get anything then you choose a teacher you can get on with and then… …then it's hard because you have to make changes. It's about changing your self. Of course the techniques and all of that you can pick up anywhere. But then to go any further than that you have to put your faith – actually I prefer not to use that word. You watch the person and you know they have integrity – and you follow – even if there are things that you feel are unusual. Because if you agree with everything that they say then you can only make a change within what your concept of the subject allows. Whereas if, when you see your teacher, you feel "I don't know what it is but this is something that I want to get" – then the process begins.

Visitor: But before that the issue is to find the teacher…that's been my biggest hurdle.

EO: Yes – but I have also spoken to many teachers – and they complain that it is so difficult to find a good student. Now, learning particular strategies or systems…you can do it. But with a particular "system" or "methodology" or "protocol" – what you are learning there is just what some other person – great or not great, as the case may be - 'tinkered' with. Now wouldn't it be wonderful if you actually learnt to become a *'tinkerer'*. If instead of learning 'strategies' you learned to become a *'strategist'*. That is the bit where you separate the one who wants to become an 'acupuncturist' and the one who wants to practice 'acupuncture'. I made a personal choice (or it was made for me) and I decided to *become* an acupuncturist. Now when people ask me, I never advise them to follow this route. Because it is so bloody hard. It is a lot easier to just say "oh I like this" or "I like that". It's up to you – you have to decide what *you* want. Whether you have this inside you or not.

…(later)…Buying that product

EO: Some visitors don't really listen. Their questions are not really questions. You have to picture where they are coming from. Before I used to get really irritated. Before that I felt constantly let down because I put faith in people. But they have every right to be who they are. And at the same time I have every right to be who I am and to answer them in the way I feel. This has helped me to graduate from the problem. Because this is a problem. Because there are a lot of unkind, cruel, selfish people that by chance or by some crooked means are in a position of power. Wherever you are – the bottom of the table or the top, if you are less immature and a little bit kinder – it's going to help. The higher up you are, the kinder and more mature you are, the more you can help people. Unfortunately in this day and age the higher up people are, more often than not, the ones who are simply after power and money. And by the very nature of their quest this almost excludes them having any kindness or maturity. That's the world we live in.

Anyway – part of it is their condition – and they are not aware of it. They want to pick and choose. It's true – they do want a really good teacher but they want to pick and choose what they learns and what they can ignore. It's like: *"I'd like to go swimming – but I don't like the water. Can we do the swimming without the water? I know it's best to do it with the water but you know...can't I get the idea about the water without going in. If I go on a course about the theory – I think there are some – then I can help others who don't like the water...But I do want to swim – I genuinely do..."*

This is what it's all about – look carefully at what is being said. These people are not being taught – they are being sold something. Even if they say they understand it... They still go and 'buy' their teachers. Well, you ain't gonna buy me. Never. Ever. Not even in your dreams.

STEALING FROM YOUR TEACHER

TS: You want me to steal from you *Sensei*?

EO: Yes..

TS: Ok – as long as I have that on record.

EO: Yes – you must have the feeling that you want to steal their knowledge. But as I said before, it is honourable theft. In truth the teacher wants you to take it too. But what I have experienced – and like that lady yesterday too – I give her a chance – I give everybody a chance... But in the long run, what is left? You , the patient – and really – just how you feel with yourself.

SH: I can see it's boiling down to that now.

EO: That's a very good term that you are using. *"Boiling Down"*. You get rid of all the other ways bit by bit. It boils down bit by bit and becomes more concentrated. And it is kind of revealed. It is pared away and you get to the core. That is absolutely right.

IT'S OK TO MAKE SOME REASONABLE MISTAKES

TS: Actually for me at the moment it is more an issue of working on my own doubts.

EO: Don't get me wrong – I doubted everything when I first started. But I don't know if it is doubt. Doubt means you are doubting yourself. I didn't doubt myself. I investigated - what I could with the tools that I had. And every time the teacher showed me something – or I learned something – I investigated it. Doubt means there is a kind of conflict in your mind. Your teacher is saying this – but you think it is something else.

TS: It's not a doubt of what the teacher is saying…

EO: I know you don't doubt me – I know that. But with the idea espoused.

TS: It's more…something happens like… I am fairly confident of my diagnosis and then…I begin to doubt whether I have picked up the right…whether I have made the right diagnosis.

EO: Well – to think that you have made the diagnosis anyway is completely wrong. What are you thinking? You don't want to think like that. You are just making the best diagnosis that you can at that time with the tools available to you and with the type of patient that is coming in. Don't think that there is a 'right' or 'wrong there'. You are doing the best one you can. And your best today will be a different best tomorrow. Then you will be able to channel your sense of doubt into improvement. Now it's actually negative. It's stopping you from improving in the way that you can. The great thing about what you are doing is that you are not going to kill anyone in the process. So go ahead and allow yourself to make some reasonable mistakes.

AN ART BEING PRACTICED SCIENTIFICALLY…

EO: I don't want you to get confused between me and *Ikeda Sensei*. I say what I say. And he says what he says. There is no contradiction. It is just that we are different people. So when you look at his stuff, don't think of me. And when you look at my stuff, don't think of him.

This is an art that is being practiced scientifically. Don't make the mistake of thinking that it is a science that it being practiced artistically. It is not. And artists must practice differently. Otherwise it is not art. In the beginning there is not so much of an art element. It is all technical specifics. But then later on there *must* be differences. If you practice the same as me then I know there is something wrong. If I practice the same as *Ikeda Sensei* then *he* knows there is something wrong. He is trying to teach us to get the basics together and then you have to form your own practice. Is that a problem for you? Don't make it a problem. Now - does this dispose of your question?

KW: He said that needling lightly mixes the *Ei Ki* (衛気; defensive *Ki*) and the *Ei Ki* (営気; nutritive *Ki*). So that healing can result. But when you treated that last patient you were just doing the surface – the *Ei Ki* (defensive *Ki*) – was there an element of the *Ei Ki* (nutritive *Ki*) also involved?

EO – Yes – did you see the surface contact needling? That was getting the *Ei Ki* (defensive *Ki*) going. But then I decided that I wanted to take this and put it in and get the *Ei Ki* (nutritive *Ki*) moving. So if you notice I didn't put the needle in quickly. I did it slowly. I feel I am kind of irritating the skin as I go in. That's where I push the *Ei Ki* (defensive *Ki*) into the inside a little bit. So you can call it "mixing" if you like. But basically as you may see I do a lot of surface needling – it's good for our health. Firstly it is defensive *Ki*. And then the other thing is I can take that, if I want, and put it in different places. So he is using the word "mixing". And he is coming from a slightly different standpoint - that of having about 20 years more experience than me.

Also I think that he is not concerned with the result. Because you know – his energy is probably a little less (but more refined) than before and when he uses it perhaps it is only when he has to rather than because he feels like it. In that respect I am still a little whipper snapper. I have a lot of energy compared to him. I remember in his younger days when I first met him – he did a lot of stuff. So that must change with time. You see – if you are in the process yourself, you can see him and understand how good he is. Most people don't have a clue. They look and they can't see. That's why I think is difficult for people to learn from him from scratch now. They are seeing the end result of many many years of practice, study and refinement. But they dont see that part

TRICKING THE BODY

EO: When we treat, we are almost trying to trick the body. We don't actually get the result of change in the body that we are looking for. What we do is to bring the pulse to where we want it – we give the patient the pulse of their healthy state. We show the body where it wants to go. Then it can get there – it knows what a good a place feels like.. This is *Ki* Medicine – we don't change the physical.

SUCCESS

EO: Sometimes success in treatment is getting the patient to lie on the couch and complain – you think it is getting them better – right?

THE TRUE VALUE OF A QUESTION

EO: The main thing is you need to try and work things out yourself before you ask a question. Sometimes when a thing is difficult to work out… it is a time when you actually learn the most. And what I'm actually saying is, not about the subject or specific thing that you are asking about.

GW: What... you learn more about yourself??

EO: No, not only about yourself, but other things too. That far outweighs the significance of your own question and answer. I give you an example.. When I was learning from *Takenouchi Sensei* at the beginning... I'd ask him a question and he'd give me five questions back. At first I didn't know what to do. I became scared to ask him a question because he would ask right there and then, what's this and what's that? So, I really wanted to ask questions...I was dying to ask a question and I would guess what kinds of questions he would ask me. So, here was my question and actually I had to study a whole lot besides. He fooled me into studying much more than I ever would have. Also, when I replied, then he gave me even more than I had expected. When he asked me a question... when I went in and asked him a question he would give me the normal run around with all the other questions and when I answered them, he then gave me some answers that I hadn`t even thought of asking for. So, actually I learnt far more than I would have even conceived of.

As I said before, if you ask a question, the only thing you can get is the answer. And if a person's ability to see or view or horizons are limited then the only thing they will get is a limited answer. So, what happens if I ask a question with a narrow frame of mind... I can't see any of the rest so that is all I can grasp. What happens if there's no question and instead I think a little bit.. When someone says something and I open up (my field of vision) and I can see a whole lot more.

The point I am making is this. The question and answer process develops to where you feel comfortable enough with the answers that I give you to relax and start learning. Not book learning. Not blinkered. It is about opening your field of vision. In my younger days I loved the question and answer routine... I still enjoy it but... they would ask this question and I would answer straight away... just like machine gun fire... it was fun but actually, when I look back I know it was no the best way to teach.

GW: I don't know how I'm ever going to be able to ask a question again!

EO: Great.

GW: But that's boring.

EO: You can ask the questions but you have to put it into context of what we are trying to do. Basically, you have to ask the questions until you are comfortable enough to really start learning.

GW: I have to ask the questions until I am comfortable enough to really start learning...?

EO: Yes. If you have to ask questions all the time, it means that you aren't ready to start learning yet. Also, I will know because the quality of the question will change. It will be much different. It will be a question after some thought. It will be a question after some looking, some observation. At the moment it's a question before thought has occurred, before observation has occurred. So, that means that you are not ready, you aren't comfortable enough yet to start looking.. to start observing, to start questioning or enquiring in a real sense. So, don't worry. I know what's going on. So you see right now I can see that you are not bothered – at this time you are too lazy to go in there.

GW: I will, I will...

EO: Do it now then. Look into it then. Think about it. In order to memorize something, what do you have to do? And what's the feeling you get when you think about all the things you have to remember...? What's the first thing that comes into your mind.

GW: めんどくさいね (tiresome/ a hassle)

EO: I rest my case. You are not alone. Everyone feels that way. But the main thing is, how much of it you can put up with in order for you to get something right. I'm different from you. Japanese wasn't my mother language, but I knew that I wanted to learn from a couple of teachers in particular and I knew that if I wanted to learn that I would have to go through the process of learning Japanese, the *kanji* etc. But that doesn't stop me from still being lazy.. it doesn't mean that I'm not lazy.. I'm saying 'OK, how much can I limit this laziness in order to get the job done'. Everybody is lazy. Everybody has a poor memory if they let it be poor.

Now, when you go though the process of actually investigating your initial question for yourself, the question will change. It's a question after consideration, a question after a lot of thought. It's a question where you actually enter into the process of enquiry. And although it's still a question, the quality is completely different. If you look at the questions we are talking about now - where the person 's question is just to get an answer so they can hopefully feel more comfortable to actually start learning… they haven't actually entered into the process of enquiry yet.

LET IT HURT!
EO: Actually we need to apply the same thinking and approach to our patients in treatment. Like the other day… I had a patient that came in and she had very bad period pain and when she got the pain she would hyper ventilate. She called up and asked for help.. but she didn't know if she could make it to the clinic. I said to her to get into a taxi and I promised her that she would get better. She came in and while I was treating her she said she felt better but that it still felt a little painful. After the treatment she went to the toilet and when she came back she said that it had completely gone!

Now, I could see what was going on.. if I had let her go home then, she would have been going away saying, "Oh, I went to the clinic and he gave me really good acupuncture and I felt so good. So in her mind she says that every time she feels pain she can come in and have acupuncture, right? That`s what most people do. It feels nice for the practitioner because she`ll say, "Oh he`s a great acupuncturist" etc. But I stopped her. I stopped that line of thinking. I said, "Well... I`m really glad you feel better but actually, I didn`t do much. All I did was to help you to relax and you got better through your own abilities. I explained to her that every time that she had her pain, she would have the pain that was occurring now, and she would also (in her mind) connect it with the pain she had had up till now. So, it was like, "Oh no! Not you again." ... that dread. And then the other thing, at the same time, she is thinking "Oh, no. If it carries on being like this... what am I going to do?" ...So, she is also extending it to the future. So, what she was doing was having one unit of pain which she was making into three units. So, tripling the effect. So, I said to her.. I always like to say this.. I said, "From now on, I want you to say, "Let it hurt!". I explained that up till now she had had that pain so many times and it didn't kill her.. she was still OK...And after a little while she was feeling OK again so there was no point in her fearing it from her past experience.

The other thing, just like *Sifu* was saying, "the pain is now.. it hasn't happened yet in the future. So, the future isn't actually there yet... The present pain... we will work on together. I will make the occurrence of the pain get less bit by bit but if you continue making it three times more powerful then it is always going to be problematic.

I explained this to her. I explained to her that with acupuncture I can make the initial pain less. I want her to do her bit too to help her get better.

So, you have to put it all into context. For her, I didn't give her just the answer that she asked for.

Her question/request was to get rid this pain. If I had done that and sent her away then every time it would happen again. That's also what treatment is all about. If we have a pain here, we don't just stick a needle here and finish, no. We don't just give them the answer to the question or the request. We give something bigger. We can make it technical and call it the root treatment or the 全身治療 (whole body treatment)。 But, it`s not just that, it`s a whole new way of looking at it. Do you see what I`m saying? This applies to many fields, obviously.

OBSERVATIONS OF THE STATE OF PRACTITIONERS

There are some people. They are so weak that when they stand, almost all the *Ki* they have is spent going inside to fill within and there`s not enough of it to go out for the patients. There are quite a few like this. Before helping others, these people have to spend some time helping themselves. From my own experience, people with weak muscles, when we get a little busy and they have a bad back, you can see they can`t give the required attention to the patient.

There`s another type who have so much *oketsu* (blood stagnation). By doing sports, they have to improve the flow in the body. The problem arises when the purpose of doing the sports becomes to get a beautiful body. When this desire becomes too strong, their purpose gets warped and instead of feeling free from their *oketsu*, instead they get obsessed with their own bodies, talk about themselves all the time… Diets too.. people who think this diet or that diet is wonderful.. they go to restaurants saying what they can't eat all the time. These people become weird after a while. These people are losing their health in the name of good health.

In conclusion, *genki*, supple, warm, sexual vitality (精力) are essential. (The reason why I included sexual vitality is that it`s part of the body`s basic energy. It doesn`t mean you have to be having sex all the time, the vitality to be able to is important.)

BURNING QUESTIONS

Q   You have mentioned that there is an optimum pulse for each person. Is there an optimum state of health for each person? Does this state of health depend on the person's environment and can a person only reach an optimum level of health if that person is in the ideal environment for him or her?

A   First, What is the ideal environment? We have to adjust our minds before we think about answering this question. In the West, we - and we all do this - tend to split mind and body. *This* question splits mind and body. It asks about physical or environmental factors, and does not take into account mental and spiritual factors. The West - and the whole world is becoming Western - often splits body and mind without even knowing it.

Now, let me ask this question. If the countryside is the best environment for a person, why would he or she move to the city? The answer is that the person had a need for some thing from the city that he or she could not get from the country. Maybe the person wanted to work or study. This "want" involves spiritual and mental aspects. If the countryside had been ideal for that person's whole health, he or she would have also been satisfied in his or her heart.

The very simple answer to the question of optimum health is that we adapt. If mental, spiritual, and physical mechanisms of our bodies are in order, then we can adapt. For instance, if I were in the Sahara desert against my will, I might have difficulty adapting on all three levels. But if I were there by choice, then, say, physically, I might have difficulty adapting, but spiritually and mentally, I would be OK. And then after some time in the desert, I would reach a state of balance in all three factors that would probably not be perfect. So we have to be very careful about the way we look at the question of health. The optimum state of health is really just a myth. Nothing is perfect.

Rather than asking about the ideal state of health, perhaps we should ask about the ideal method of adapting. This question is interesting. The answer is that adapting is a crooked path. Part of the adaption process involves being on-course; the other part is going off-course. We might be on-course for a time, then we go off, and then we go on-course again. Despite the digressions, progress is there - we continue to move forward.

When I was a child, I was interested in outer space. One thing I always remember from the first Apollo mission is that scientists said the Apollo was off-course 90% of the time. Yet it *still* got to the moon. This was an important lesson for me. You do not have to be straight on-course all the time. Knowing this takes the pressure off when working towards our goals, whether we are going to the moon, wanting a good relationship, trying to be healthy - anything. We do not have to be perfect. You can be 90% off-course, or more but you can achieve your goals as long as your adaptive mechanisms are in place. And this is where acupuncture, herbal medicine, and other natural medical systems are strong.

Regarding treatment, you can also go off-course. Sometimes you improve someone's health to a certain level, but sometimes you make them a little bit worse. When you realise a digression has ocurred, you swing the patient back the other way. You adapt. When you get better at treating, the margin of error becomes smaller.

So you must not think that you are going to treat someone without making mistakes. You must not approach a problem saying, "OK. I am not going to make a mistake." This is not the right attitude—it is a negative one. This approach is like driving with the handbrake on in hopes of preventing an accident. You are resisting. So just try to do your best. You can make mistakes. You may regret making a mistake, but you will improve because of it. Work on the adapting and the goals will fall into place.

CHAPTER 2

Needling

2.1 THE NEEDLING TRUTH

Amongst those of us practising acupuncture and moxibustion, many have misconceptions about what a needle is. A needle today is usually used for straight insertion, but as I've mentioned in seminars and study groups over the years, a needle around the time of the Yellow Emperor's Inner Classic (黃帝內經, *Huangdi Neijing*) was something qualitatively different. Recently, I visited an old friend of mine in Hawaii (if you're going to visit someone, for God's sake, make sure the person lives in Hawaii) who's a professor of Chinese philosophy. Amongst his many accomplishments, he's still able to make an English breakfast consisting of bacon and eggs with the black bits sticking to the latter. Where these black bits come from—and indeed, where they go—are certainly questions that demand answering, but not here and not now.

Anyway, during one of our discussions, I asked him what philosophy actually was. He took my question in stride, answering very simply that to him it was the prerequisite for all other studies. Study can begin once an initial approach, method of thinking or, dare I say, "philosophy," is in place.

I remember thinking at the time about the practice of Oriental medicine in general, and as I'm fond of saying recently, acupuncture—and moxibustion in particular—is the medicine of nothing. That is to say, from a piece of metal and a wad of moxa, we create a therapy that deals with all manners of ailments. But we can't treat with just metal and moxa. It's imperative that we have the software, the insides, the philosophy that animates Oriental medicine. Unfortunately, the software is often not in place, as can be seen when a practitioner's idea of a needle is no different from that of the patient.

We should have a look at what the Yellow Emperor's Inner Classic has to say. The very first chapter of the *Ling Shu* (靈枢; *Rei Su* in Japanese; translated as the "Spiritual Pivot") (one of two parts of the Yellow Emperor) is the "Nine Needles and Twelve Origins" (九鍼十二原) and gives us important information on how the ancient Chinese viewed needles. As I'll demonstrate, the ancient views are actually vastly different from the views held by most acupuncturists today.

This first chapter of the *Ling Shu* is such a superb one that I really should translate all of it because it gives us the first images of needling that we should hold in our minds and hearts as we start (or continue) our study and practice of this precious art. Oh well, having said all this, I suppose I should translate the chapter for you. It's rather long, so I might skip a few bits here and there. Forgive me.

NINE NEEDLES AND TWELVE ORIGINS (九鍼十二原)

Let's begin with our first excerpt.

黄帝問於歧伯曰：余子萬民，養百姓而收其租稅；
余哀其不給而屬有疾病。余欲勿使被毒藥，無用砭
石，欲以微鍼通其經脈，調其血氣，榮其逆順出入
之會。令可傳於後世，必明為之法，令終而不滅，
久而不絕，易用難忘，為之經紀，異其章，別其表
裏，為之終始。令各有形，先立鍼經。願聞其情。

The Yellow Emperor enquired of the physician, "I consider the people to be my children, and I help the common people and receive their tribute. However, I'm sometimes lacking and my beloved people suffer from a multitude of diseases. I would like them to stop using ineffective and possibly harmful poison compresses and stone lancets. Rather, I would prefer that they utilize the delicate, painless needling system to regulate the Blood and Ki in the meridians and ensure the smooth and orderly flow of these in the organism. This system should be preserved for future generations, its methods illuminated, ensuring that it will not die or diminish. It is a system that is easy to use and difficult to forget. I want to detail the authentic methods in an ordered fashion, distinguishing between the exterior and interior with no omissions. I want to detail all that is necessary for those who want to practice true acupuncture. Please physician, instruct me as to the finer points of the art."

歧伯答曰：臣請推而次之，令有綱紀，始於一，終
於九焉。

The physician, Gihaku, replied, "Very well, my Lord. I will do what you have requested. It will consist of nine sections."

That the Yellow Emperor preferred delicate, painless needling to harmful compresses and stone lancets is to be expected, but if we look carefully at his words, we can also discern that he's asking for a different way to treat disease. He's asking us to favour tonifcation (working not on the disease, but on the person, i.e., the meridians) rather than concentrating on dispersion (working on the disease by expelling it by poisoning or lancing). Also, he's making it clear that needling using a delicate, painless method is for regulating the Blood and *Ki* of the meridians and that needles are not just to be bunged in here and there without consideration.

Although the Yellow Emperor says he received tribute (normally about 10 percent of agricultural production) from the common people, he was (is), as far as I remember, unusual in that there were no sacrifices made to him. Most other gods or god-like figures were given sacrifices, but the Yellow Emperor was considered to be in a special category. There are even those now who consider him too have been an extraterrestrial.. The following bit was said by *Gihaku*.

九鍼之玄要在終始。故能知終始、一言而畢。不知
終始。鍼道成絶。

The subtle importance of the Nine Needles lies in the mechanism of form and potential. If there is knowledge of form and potential, the art can be comprehended in one word. If there is a lack of knowledge of this, the way of acupuncture will be lost. [13]

The physician is telling us that we need a prerequisite for understanding or practising acupuncture. We get the idea of prerequisite from the

---

[13] This particular passage is included in *Shibasaki's* version of the *Ling Shu*. It does not appear in other versions that I have checked. I like it though and I will leave it in.

words that I translated as "form and potential" and that are represented by the characters 終 and, 始 respectively. Nowadays, these characters usually mean "finish" and "start." The ancient meanings of these two words, however, are more along the lines of "fullness or completion" and "beginning or birth."

I guess what we are talking about is the mechanism behind two opposite phenomena, which we could call the mechanism behind *Yin* and *Yang*. (In English, we might say "the ins and outs" off a subject.) Anyway if this is the case, I'm wondering why these characters and were used and not the characters for *Yin* and *Yang*. The point I really want to make is that a prerequisite is needed, a philosophy for making sense of and practising true acupuncture according to the classics. So my friend in Hawaii was right!

"Form and potential "終始" is the mechanism behind the basic functions of the universe. These functions are those that produce form or fullness as well as the potential for creativity or birth. When the practitioner has knowledge of this, he or she is meshed with the universe, and in the context of the universe, the disease of the patient is a mere dot of a phenomenon—and a mere dot can be easily overcome. When the patient can also mesh with the universe, we're talking about rapid recovery of any disease!

So *Gihaku's* words are challenging us: Do we have even an inkling of the workings of the universe? Can we move beyond the normal, conditioned mind-set of disease and health, patient and practitioner, them and us? But don't worry, my friends. Even if we can achieve a greater awareness of how a patient thinks, lives and works, this awareness will be a step forward in performing true acupuncture[14]. Of

---

[14] So for instance, if a patient is known to be a busy executive who's involved in negotiations and quick decision-making and who plays and works hard, this patient has to be considered and treated in light of these factors. Translated into clinical detail, we can say that at the very least, this patient will probably function better in a *Yin* deficient state. Thus, even if this patient presents with what appears to be a mildly deficient

course, if we really get it together, there's a strong possibility we'll have a religion named after us—or at least an airport or a few buildings.

Anyway, *Gihaku* continues:

請言其道！小鍼之要，易陳而難入。麤守形，上守神。神乎神，客在門。未覩其疾，惡知其原？刺之微在速遲。麤守關，上守機，機之動，不離其空。

The importance of the way of delicate needling is easy to speak about but difficult to practice. The technician is concerned with form; the master physician is concerned with shen. The shen and pathogenic Ki can be found in the gates [points]. When there are still no symptoms present, how can the source [of the disease] be known?

空中之機，清靜而微。其來不可逢，其往不可追。知機之道者，不可掛以發。不知機道，扣之不發。知其往來，要與之期。麤之闇乎，妙哉，工獨有之。

The finesse or subtlety of needling is to be found in the speed or slowness of use. The technician is concerned about physical check areas of the body; the master physician is concerned with the stirrings of action within the body, the movement that can be observed through the acupuncture points. The presence of this stirring of action in the points is pure, still and delicate in nature. The arrival must not be met and its going must not be followed. The person who knows about the stirrings of action does not leave a gap off even a

pulse and abdomen, he should be treated for *Yang* deficiency to deliberately put him into a Yin deficient state. Even this small change from the norm for this type of patient couldn't have been conceived of if the practitioner didn't have the ability to see beyond the normal state of affairs.

single hair's breadth when needling. The person that is unaware of the stirrings of action misses the correct opportunity to needle.

往者為逆，來者為順，明知逆順，正行無問。迎而奪之，惡得無虛？追而濟之，惡得無實？迎之隨之，以意和之，鍼道畢矣。

Knowledge of the arrival and going [of the Ki and Blood] is important because it gives us the timing. The technician is not illuminated by this knowledge; only the master physician has this sense. The going [fading of Ki and Blood] is known as disorderly [perversion] and the arrival [forming] is known as orderly [correct]. If there is a clear knowledge of disorderly and orderly movement, appropriate treatment can be carried out with no doubts whatsoever. Why does whittling down the perversion not lead to deficiency? Why does following and increasing not lead excess? When meeting or following, the mind must be in harmony. This is the general guide to the way of acupuncture.

In the above excerpt, *Gihaku* talks of the master practitioner being concerned with *shin* (神 ; Spirit). If there's observation (and understanding) of *shin*, there's an automatic understanding of the absence or presence of *Ki*, Blood and Fluids of the patient, i.e., the patient's energetics rather than just the physical factors. Further down the passage *Gihaku* says that the technician concerned with physical check areas. For instance, practitioners who find tender points on the abdomen, then needle a point (usually distally), and come back to check the tenderness are primarily concerned with the physical.

This is not to say that this method of working has no merit; rather, we should realise that this is an intermediate stage in a practitioner's development; it's not mastery. But the intermediate stage is a necessary precursor for the higher stage, where energy (the presence or lack of it) is mainly considered. I'd like to point out one more bit from the previous passage. When *Gihaku* says that the *"arrival must not be met and its going must not be followed,"* he means that the practitioner must remain neutral and not overreact.

Well, enough of that. Here's another bit.

> 凡用鍼者，虛則實之，滿則泄之，宛陳則除之，邪勝則虛之。大要曰：徐而疾則實，疾而徐則虛。
>
> *Those who practice the art of acupuncture should fill the deficiencies and deflate the areas that are tight and full. Old, stagnant Blood should be removed. If pathogenic Ki is dominant, there is deficiency. In general terms, for excess conditions, the method should be slow and then fast. For deficiency, it should be fast and then slow.*

The passage above talks about removing old, stagnant Blood. For a more in-depth look at bloodletting, or micro-bleeding, please see "Principles of Acupuncture and Moxibustion in the Yellow Emperor" and "Commentary on *Shibasaki's* translation" in *A Long Road* (Volume III); Chapter 2.

Also in the last passage, *Gihaku* describes needling methods. For excess conditions, the insertion needs to be slow to scrape the Defensive (*Yang*) *Ki* and gather the pathogenic *Ki* around the needle. Withdrawal should be fast, having the feeling of taking away something. For deficiency, the insertion needs to be fast to avoid injuring the Defensive (*Yang*) *Ki*, and the withdrawal should be done slowly to achieve the feeling of leaving something behind.

Here's another section from the chapter:

言實與虛，若有若無。察後與先。若存若亡。為虛
與實，若得若失。虛實之要，九鍼最妙，補寫之
時，以鍼為之。寫曰，必持內之，放而出之，排陽
得鍼，邪氣得泄。按而引鍼，是謂內溫，血不得
散，氣不得出也。補曰，隨之隨之，意若妄之。若
行若按，如蚊虻止，如留如還，去如弦絕，令左屬
右，其氣故止，外門已閉，中氣乃實，必無留血，
急取誅之。

Talking of excess and deficiency is like [talking of] something and nothing. Or it is like examining something from behind and the front. Or it is like existence or non-existence. By acting on [with tonification and shunting] deficiency and excess, there will be a corresponding gain or loss. Understanding the importance of deficiency and excess represents the most sublime level of the nine needles method. When needling deficiency, tonify. For excess, you must shunt. For shunting, hold [the needle] firmly and still [with the left hand]. Gather [the Ki] and release it. Make a gap in the Yang Ki and let the pathogenic Ki gathered beneath the needle leak out. If the left hand is pressed when the needle is withdrawn, it leads to a condition known as Heat Stagnation trapped inside, which means that the pathogenic Blood and Ki can not be released.

Tonification means "to follow," and the meaning of follow is "to abandon yourself and your own ideas." Move smoothly without hesitation, pressing very smoothly. It must be like a mosquito or a gadfly alighting [on the skin], stopping or moving. Leaving should be like cutting a thread, withdrawing with the right hand while the left hand stays glued to the point,

> *stopping any leakage of Ki. The point should be closed, allowing the Ki inside to become full. Blood that has become stagnant should be removed.*

In the above passage, regarding the condition "*Heat Stagnation trapped inside*" *Gihaku* appears to be telling us not to press when shunting, as this may lead to a feeling of something added or gained, thus leading to tonification of the pathogen.

Further down the section *Gihaku* describes the meaning of "following." Here we have the same mind-set and principles as things Taoist. I can't help feeling I'm reading about push hands in *Tai Chi*.

In the next passage, *Gihaku* further describes the way of needling.

持鍼之道，堅者為寶。正指直刺，無鍼左右。神在
秋毫，屬意病者。審視血脈者，刺之無殆。方刺之
時，必在懸陽，及與兩衛。神屬勿去，知病存亡。
血脈者在俞橫居，視之獨澄，切之獨堅。

In order to follow the way of acupuncture, there must be a state of spiritual tension. The needle should be inserted straight in with no wavering to the left or right. The practitioner must be thorough and delicate and become one with the patient. The blood vessels should be examined in a detailed fashion. If these are needled, there will be no regrets. When needling, practitioners should have their mind on the two Defensive Ki's. If the spirit is concentrated, the absence or presence of disease [sites] can be known. Blood vesselss [for micro-bleeding] are located around [not on] the acupuncture points. These will be clearly seen as independent, raised areas [of Blood], and when touched, they will feel taut and different from the surrounding areas.

Gihaku talks here of the need for spiritual tension. When needling is gentle, the inside (spirit) must be very firm and unyielding, almost relentless in nature. When needling is strong, the spirit must be gentle and compassionate. There's a saying that needling should be performed as if "holding down the tiger." This should not be mistaken to mean we should grip the needle with physical strength (This would only inhibit the flow of *Ki*). Rather, the saying is alluding to the spiritual state connected with doing this needling. The two Defensive *Ki*'s (兩衛) have been variously translated as Defensive *Ki* of the outside the body (circulating outside the skin or the Earth, for instance) and as Defensive *Ki* of the inside the body (of the *Zang* organs or the area between the eyebrows, for example).

I'm afraid I beg to differ with these interpretations. I believe that the practitioner has to mesh the patient and him or herself with the universe. This is done through an exchange between the Defensive *Ki* of the body and that of the earth. This type of concept is made use of in *Zhiineng Chi kung* (知能気功) and is known as H*ui Yuan Chi* (混元気). If the mind is on the Defensive *Ki* of both the patient the earth (taken as the image of the horizon), the *Ki* of the universe can be more easily utilised to bring about a cure. Thinking of the mind as being confined only to the patient encourages the mistaken and actually quite prevalent view that the body (and thus the healing event) is an isolated mechanism from the universe.

Now in the nextsection, *Gihaku* starts to describe the classical Nine Needles.

九鍼之名，各不同形。一曰鑱鍼，長一寸六分；二曰員鍼，長一寸六分；三曰鍉鍼，長三寸半；四曰鋒鍼，長一寸六分；五曰鈹鍼，長四寸，廣二分半；六曰員利鍼，長一寸六分；七曰毫鍼，長三寸六分；八曰長鍼，長七寸；九曰大鍼，長四寸。

The nine needles have differing names and shapes. The first is called the Zan needle. It is 1 cun, 6 bun long. The second [needle] is called the En needle. It is 1 cun, 6 bun long. The third is called the Tei needle. It is 3-and-a-half cun in length. The fourth is called the Ho needle. It is 1 cun, 6 bun long. The fifth is thee Hi needle. It is 4 cun long and 2- and-a-half bun wide. The sixth is the En ri needle. It is 1 cun, 6 bun long. The seventh is the Go needle and it is 3 cun, 6 bun in length. The eighth is the Cho needle, which is 7 cun in length. The ninth is the Dai needle, which is 4 cun in length.

The *Zan* (鑱) needle can be translated as "thin, fitting needle," and the *En* (員) needle can bet translated as "round needle." The *Tei* (鍉) needle can be translated as "arrow-point needle", the *Ho* (鋒) needle as "three-edged needle" and the *Hi* (鈹) needle as "knife-needle." The *En Ri* (員利) needle can be translated as "round, sharp needle." The *Go* (毫) needle can be translated as "long, delicate needle," the *Cho* (長) needle as "long needle," and the *Dai* (大) needle as "big needle."

As can be seen by looking at the sizes, no needle is shorter than 1 cun, 6 bun, and the longest is 7 cun. In modern times, the average needle length used is often 1 cun, 3 bun (or less). Also of note is that the needle said to resemble the most often-used needle of today, the *Go* needle, was in fact 3 cun, 6 bun in length, which actually puts this needle in the longer range, with longer needles between 4 and 7 cun in length.

Next, *Gihaku* explains the special characteristics and uses of the needles.

鑱鍼者，頭大末銳，去寫陽氣
The Zan needle has a large head and a sharp point and is used to shunt the Yang Ki.
員鍼者，鍼如卵形，揩摩分間，不得傷肌肉，以寫分氣；

The En needle is shaped like an egg and is used to rub in between the connective tissues without harming the flesh. It shunts the Ki that is trapped there.

鍉鍼者，鋒如黍粟之銳，主按脈勿陷，以致其氣；

The Tei needle has a point that is shaped like a millet seed and is used to press or massage blood vessels, but is not used to pierce them. It is used to improve the flow of Ki throughout the body.

鋒鍼者，刃三隅以發痼疾，

The Ho needle has a three-edged point and is used for chronic diseases.

鈹鍼者，末如劍鋒，以取大膿；

The point of the Hi needle is shaped like a sword and is used to remove pus from the body.

員利鍼者，大如氂，且員且銳，中身微大，以取暴氣

The En ri needle is as thin as a hair and the tip is round but sharp. The shaft of the needle is slightly larger [slightly wider than the tip]. It is used for acute diseases.

毫鍼者，尖如蚊虻喙，靜以徐往，微以久留之而養，以取痛痺

The Go needle has a point shaped like the proboscis of a mosquito or a gadfly. It is inserted slowly, bit by bit, and left in place, nourishing thee area and eliminating pain and numbness.

長鍼者，鋒利身薄，可以取遠痺

The Cho needle has a sharp point and a thin shaft and is used for chronic numbness.

大鍼者，尖如梃，其鋒微員，以寫機關之水也。

> *The Dai needle is like straight stick with a small, round tip and is used to shunt watery [waterlogged] areas around the hips.*
>
> 九鍼畢矣。
>
> *This is the end of the explanation of the nine needles.*

It's also the end of my translation! At this juncture, I'd like to pose a question: How many of the above needles are for straight insertion?

MORE ABOUT THE NEEDLES
Zan（鑱）*needling*

The *Zan* needle can be thought of as similar to the *Yoneyama*-type *hifu shin* (skin needle), which is shaped like a shark's fin and is used to briskly rub, vibrate and scrape the skin. This leaves the skin a little red and shunts the *Yang Ki*. I use it for shunting *Yang Ki* at the *Tai Yang* level, too be precise.

If you want to go deeper than this, you have to change to another tool to avoid causing damage to the skin and flesh.

En（員）*Needling*

If the *Zan* needle is useful for clearing Heat at the *Tai Yang* level, then the *En* needle is the one for clearing Heat from the *Yang Ming*. This needle is one of my favourites, and I use it when I want to shunt Heat that is stuck in connective tissues of the ankles, knees (I leave the hips to the *Dai* needle), wrists, elbows, shoulders, neck and especially the inner scapular regions. I tend to use it with a cream to avoid damaging the flesh (as the above translated passage on *En* needling tells us) and to allow better movement along the tight areas. In this way, I'm able to distinguish clearly between the *Tai Yang* level (involving mostly the skin) and the *Yang Ming* level (by-passing the skin and going deeper into the body).

Tei (鍉) *needling*

This type of needling is very good for *Yang* deficient patients, or conversely, patients with very heavy Blood Stagnation. I had a phase where I almost exclusively used the *Tei* needle for all of my root treatments. You could perhaps call this "touch-needling." I found that the thickness of the *Tei* needle seemed to make this needle more effective than an ordinary 1-cun, 3-bun, zero-gauge needle. When I used it for *Yang* Deficiency treatments, I was—without really thinking about it—using points on or very near blood vessels. Good examples of such points include *Tai En* (太淵; LU9), *Tai Kei* (太谿; KI3) and *Sho Yo* (衝陽; ST42). Needling these points with a *Tei* needle had a very good effect without any wastage of *Yang Ki*. A copper or gold *Tei* needle appeared to be the best. The point of this needling is that we utilise the blood vessels. In some cases, I used the blood vessel system to sort of bypass the meridian system when I felt it was too clogged up. This clogging often occurs with heavy Blood Stagnation. In cases like these, I use a 1-cun, 3-bun, zero-gauge needle or a 1-cun, 6-bun, one-gauge needle to needle one or any combination of *Tai En* (LU9), *Reku Ketsu* (列欸; LU7) (but taking it smack on the artery) and *Tai Kei* (KI3). For *Tai Kei*, I actually insert the needles (one in each leg) until their tips are resting on the arteries, producing a noticeable twitch that could be seen moving in time to the heartbeat. The needles are left in place for 15 to 20 minutes, resulting in quite a deep tonification of the system.

Ho (鋒) *needling*

This type of needling is basically bloodletting (micro-bleeding). The nearest equivalent to this needle nowadays in Japan is the *San Ryo Shin* (三稜鍼), literally the "three-edged needle."

Hi (鈹) *needling*

This type of needling is the equivalent of using a scalpel to remove pus from the body. I don't have much experience with this except for one case I remember, when I lanced a huge boil that was sitting on the upper part of the Governor vessel.

En Ri (員利) *needling*

An *En Ri* needle has a ring at one end and a sharp point at the other. It can be used to brush the skin with the former and lightly prick the skin with the latter. The *Ling Shu* says it was used for acute diseases, so it was probably use to clear Heat from the *Tai Yang* (the most exterior) part of the body. It was therefore likely used in a lighter way than, for example, the *En* needle.

Go (毫) *needling*

The *Go* needle is long and thin and most resembles the type of needle in use today, but with some differences. According to the *Ling Shu*, we know that it's one of the longer needles in the repertoire and that it's tonifying in nature. We can infer its tonifying nature because the description of the *Go* needle that I translated above uses the characters 蚊 and 虻 , meaning mosquito and gadfly respectively, which connects this section with an earlier section I translated that mentioned both "tonification" and "mosquitos and gadflys alighting (in a way that they cannot be felt) on the skin."

Regarding the usage of the *Go* needle, the last passage I translated says that the needles should be inserted and left in place. If the needles are to be inserted, then they should be inserted very shallowly. Thinking about this, I recalled a senior fellow-student of mine who insisted on using longer needles, despite only just breaking the skin with extremely light surface-needling. He said he did this because the longer needles caused *Yang Ki* to collect more heavily. In thinking about how to explain this phenomenon, I was forced to come up with the term "antenna effect." That is to say, the long needle acts as a sort of antenna through which matter, energy and information, i.e., *Ki* can be picked up and gathered into the body. This *Ki* is not just the body's *Ki*. Because of the length of the needle, it draws from the environment, the universe if you will. We could propose that the longer the needle, the greater the amount of *Ki* that can be gathered from the universe.

It may seem paradoxical that with this longer needle, we must needle more shallowly than usual. We must also keep our minds less on the *Yin* insides of the body and more on the gathering of *Yang Ki* from outside the body. This will mesh the patient with the rest of the universe and discourage the "isolated unit" tendency so common amongst practitioners.

It is interesting to note that when I first opened my clinic, I used very short 1-cun needles, and over time, I stepped up the size to 1-cun, 3-bun needles. Recently, I've been experimenting with 1-cun, 6-bun needles—with startling results. I've been using these needles with *Yang* deficient patients, needling them on the back-*Shu* points[15]. I insert the needles extremely shallowly so that they just about stay in, then leave them in place for a little longer than usual, about 15 to 25 minutes.

The great thing about using these longer needles is that you naturally need fewer needles for each patient, which is in itself tonifying. I generally need a maximum of six needles on the back, with four needles often being sufficient. Using these needles has produced extremely good results. Nearly all patients treated with this type of needling (including experienced acupuncturists) feel an increased sense of warmth and relaxation all over. Please try it for yourself! As a matter of interest, I also tried the same needles with a slightly deeper insertion (to a total depth of 1 to 2 mm), which appeared to have absolutely no effect whatsoever.

---

[15] Remember that the back-*shu* (*shu* meaning "to transport or communicate") points are being used here to have an effect, not just within the body between different organs, but between the body and the universe. For a more in-depth discussion of the back-*shu* points, please see "Commentary on *Shibasaki's* Translation," A Long Road, Volume III, Chapter 2

Cho (長) *needling*

This type of needling is one of the more robust types of needling (the *Cho* needle being the longest of the Nine Needles) often performed by Chinese-style practitioners.

Dai (大) *needling*

I reserve this type of needling for the buttocks, not just because of the reference to it in the *Ling Shu*, but because of the sheer stimulus it provides. On a normal-sized person, the buttocks are about the only place this type of needle could be gainfully employed. The buttocks have huge, powerful muscles that contain a lot of Blood, and therefore, a lot of Water. Also, the buttocks represent a large part of the lower Heater, so stimulating them will clear unwanted Water or Fluid from the body. In my student days, I knew a practitioner who treated every patient, no matter what the problem, in the buttocks. At that time, the incredibly loud snoring of one of my classmates came to the attention of this practitioner. After examining my classmate, he declared that the snoring was caused by Fluid Stagnation. He duly treated my friend in the buttocks, who reported a very deep pressure sensation in his entire buttocks, lower abdomen and lower back.

After the treatment, my classmate went to the toilet many times, and that night, as witnessed by his wife, the snoring completely stopped - only to return the next day even louder than before, after which his wife forbad him to have any more treatments. But I concluded, even at that time, that deep, strong needling to the buttocks seemed to powerfully move the Fluids.

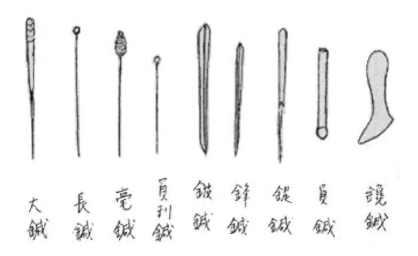

Figure 2-1: The Nine Needles

From left to right: *Dai* (big needle); *Cho* (long needle); *Go* (long, delicate needle); *En Ri* (round, sharp needle); *Hi* (knife needle); *Ho* (three-edged needle); *Tei* (arrow-point needle); *En* (round needle); *Zan* (thin, fitting needle).

The thing I dislike about this type of discussion is that it normally ends like a whiff of perfume, nice-smelling, but only giving a taste of what is to come. Well, here are some case histories to demonstrate a few applications of the Nine Needles.

CASE HISTORIES
Case one: Zan （鑱） *needling*

A foreign physiotherapist with a strong interest in acupuncture visited my clinic to observe me at work. She was very polite, but expressed doubt about the efficiency of *Zan* needle methods, implying that only deep, strong needling could be of use for pain syndromes or those involving lack of mobility. I smiled and asked her if she would like to make a small bet. She also smiled and said that she had been suffering from sciatica of her left leg and was experiencing pain from the buttock down to the foot. The pain was such that she was unable to bend forward from the waist to touch her toes.

It's funny how medical professionals (I include acupuncturists as well) can sometimes use their medical knowledge to great disadvantage for both themselves and their patients. This physiotherapist was no exception, I learned, as she explained to me, whilst preparing to be treated, the reasons why she wouldn't get any benefit from the treatment she was about to receive. I did the only sensible thing at the time: I agreed with her.

Then I proceeded with the treatment, having her lay on her side with left buttock and leg facing upwards. I examined her and found the area around *Sho Fu* (承扶; BL36) to be extremely tight. I took out my *Yoneyama*-type shark fin and began to vibrate and move the muscular tissues of the buttocks and upper thigh with butterfly-like speed and rhythm. With each sweep of the needle, I made sure it caught on the hard area around *Sho Fu* (BL36). Bit by bit, the area loosened up. Then I had her bring her knee closer to her chest before repeating the butterfly maneuvers. After about 15 minutes, her knee was comfortably up to her chest. I finished off the treatment, then asked her to bend down to test her leg, which she did. She touched her toes and came up a believer.

Case two: En (員) needling

A 72-year-old male with severe lower-back pain. The patient had been suffering for three weeks with severe lower-back pain so that sleep was disturbed and that sitting for any length of time was impossible. He had caught a cold a week or so before the onset of the lower-back pain. Thirty years earlier, he had surgery for a herniated disc.

He was wearing a corset, was of a relatively strong constitution and had a hacking cough that was worse at night. He had a strong build, his ear lobes were larger than usual and his tongue had a white coating. The lower abdomen was a little flaccid, with a little bit of tension just below the rib cage. The pulse was very weak and slow overall, with some tightness. The left-proximal and left-medial pulses were particularly deficient.

The patient was treated for Liver *Yang* Deficiency. The tight pulse may have been due to pain, but the presence of slowness suggested Cold. The white tongue confirmed the presence of Cold. Touch-needling was performed on the abdomen. *Tai Kei* (KI3) and *Tai Sho* (LV3) were tonified, and needles were retained very superficially on the painful areas of the back. Moxibustion was performed sparingly to the lower abdomen (*Chu Jo Ryu Kyu* or triangle-*kyu*[16]) and on the lower back.

The above treatment was performed three times over an interval of ten days. The patient reported that he felt great relief from pain. His pulse was stronger and quicker, and his abdomen had become less flaccid. However, the patient was still wearing the corset and the area around the lower back felt stiff to the touch.

I questioned the patient in a more detailed fashion as to the condition of his back. From this, I learned he was pain free all of the time, except when he coughed. The action of coughing caused intense pain in his lower back, which made him unable to relax. I realised from this that I had to treat the cough to clear the back problem. I wanted to use the fourth session to work only on the cough, so after taking time to convince the patient of this (After all, he came in to have his back treated), I switched gears and treated him for Liver *Yin* Deficiency with Lung Heat. His pulse was stronger than before, so I had no doubts that a *Yin* Deficiency treatment would be okay. *Fuku Ryu* (KI7) and *Chu Ho* (中封; LV4) were tonified, whilst the Lung Heat was shunted with a simple insertion to *Ko Sai* (孔最; LU6). Lastly, *Gyo Sai* (魚際; LU10) was tonified.

---

[16] See Article 4.1 entitled "Two Sides of a Moxibustion Coin".

The patient was then turned over, and I could see that the Heat was trapped deep in the muscles of the upper back. *Chi Netsu Kyu* (heat perception moxibustion[17]) on its own was not going to be enough to get in there, so I chose to use the *En* needle, with Purple Cloud ointment as the lubricant, to rub deep into the area between the shoulder blades. This caused the whole area to become red. Then one round of *Chi Netsu Kyu* was applied to the harder points, and we finished the treatment. That evening, the patient called me, saying that he had stopped coughing and felt really good. Three days later, the patient came in for another treatment with his wife—and was corset-less, cough-less and completely pain free. Examination of the lower back showed it to be relaxed with a healthy tonus.

Case three: Tei (鍉) needling

A 30-year-old female patient came to see me when my clinic was full. She had come in, not for a treatment, but to collect an herbal prescription that was to help her with her energy level. I asked her a few questions, just to make some last minute checks to see if the decoction I was thinking of was the correct one. She complained of having a fever that day, and from the pulse, it appeared that she was Lung deficient, with Heat stuck in the *Yang Ming* meridians and at the *Yang Ming* level. I realised then that the herbal decoction that was targeting her appetite, energy and constitution in general, was not right for her whilst she had the cold. The clinic was full, so I had a choice: give her another herbal decoction such as *Kakkon To* (葛根湯; *Ge Gen Tang*) or *Peuraria* Decoction—or do something else.

I suddenly remembered the gold *Tei* needle in my pocket, so I decided to treat her in the waiting room. Finding the dent at *Tai En* (LU9), I searched for the artery very carefully. I pressed the needle very lightly onto the artery, fixing it in position with my left hand, concentrating on the artery, rather than the point or the meridian. The patient said she felt

---

[17] See Article 3.1 entitled "Introduction to Moxibustion".

a deep sensation of something moving along her hand and arm. I repeated the procedure on the other side, with similar results.

I was then called into the clinic and was busy for five minutes. The patient then called out from the waiting room, saying that she had begun to sweat profusely. I got one of my assistants to give her a towel so that she could dry herself down in the toilet. Another five minutes passed with me busy treating another patient. I returned to the waiting room to find her feeling much better. The feeling of fever had disappeared.

I then gave the original herbal decoction and said that she could probably start it the next day if the cold went away. She called the next day to say that everything was fine and that she had begun taking the decoction. So this result appears to be in line with the words of the *Ling Shu* I translated earlier that talked of using the *Tei* needle to improve the flow of *Ki* throughout the body.

Incidentally, I also tried *Tei* needling on other patients with *Yin* Deficiency Syndromes to little or no effect.

Case four: Ho (鋒) *needling*

For case histories on *Ho* needling, or bloodletting, please refer to "Principles of the Yellow Emperor at work" in A Long Road (Volume III), Chapter 2.

Case five: Go (毫) *needling*

A tired, 40-something male acupuncturist was suffering from tiredness and the beginnings of a slight cold. Being an acupuncturist meant this person was one of the worst types of patients. He was so busy that he never left enough time for a full treatment.

He was of medium build and had a slightly white tongue. The pulse was slightly weak, especially in the left-distal and right-medial positions.

Because the patient was so busy, he simply had four 1-cun, 6-bun, two-gauge needles inserted to a depth of 0.1 mm and left in place for 15 minutes. The results were surprising—even for this patient who had had experience receiving and applying a large number of therapeutic modalities. He reported feeling a greater sense of relaxation, sooner than with the usual type of needling. In fact, he reported he was so relaxed that he felt as if the weight of his body was going to break the bed! This patient was me, and the types of sensations I felt were mirrored by many other patients.

Case six: Dai (大) needling

A forty-eight-year old housewife suffering from a runny nose and sore throat The patient had been successfully treated by me for glaucoma. She had been to her doctor who said that she had a cold. After two weeks of the same symptoms, she believed that she had not a cold, but perhaps an allergy.

She had a large build, was overweight, and had larger-than-normal lips and eyes. The tongue showed nothing unusual. The pulse was sunken and rough all over. It was especially deficient in the left-distal and right-medial positions. The left-medial pulse was sunken and in excess.

The patient was treated for Spleen Deficiency Liver Excess using *Dai Ryo* (PC7), *Tai Haku* (SP3) plus *Sho Yo* (ST42) for the water retention. The Liver Excess was shunted using *Yo Ryo Sen* (GB34). Needles were retained on the back for fifteen minutes at a very shallow depth.

Lastly, the patient was needled on the left and right buttocks at *Sho Fu* (BL36) using the Dai needle. The patient felt a deep squeezing sensation from this needle in the buttocks and lower back. I deliberately resisted the temptation to needle the *Yang Ming* meridians, preferring to see if I could resolve the problem just through moving the Blood and Fluids. The patient telephoned the next day with some interesting information: Not only were her nose and throat somewhat better, but also her feet weren't as swollen. She remarked that on her way to the clinic before the treatment, her shoes had felt tight, but on the way back, they felt almost loose on her feet.

This patient's larger-than-normal lips indicated a Spleen Deficient Stomach Heat constitution, whilst the relatively large eyes indicated Liver Excess. The runny nose and very sunken pulse indicated Damp, which clogged up the whole system. Upon being questioned, the patient revealed that she consumed large portions of fruit daily. Normally, I'd have used the *Yang Ming* meridians, but in this case, I was determined to focus the treatment on moving the Fluids. It appears that using the Dai needle on the buttocks and hips can be very effective for moving trapped Fluids out of the body.

2.2   ABDOMINAL & BACK RETAINED NEEDLING

TS: *Sensei*, when you go for the abdominal points, are you expecting to find hard areas there or are you going there because it is particular points which you are looking to utilise?

EO: It is a mixture of both of these. The truth is I go where my hand takes me. But I am of course informed by my knowledge. So, I go there based on a mixture of my knowledge and my feelings at the time determined by the circumstances and the other information I have been exposed to in relation to the patient. But of course, if I don't find hardness, then I don't do *Chi Shin* (置鍼; retained needling) there. And therefore we would not expect to be doing *Chi Netsu Kyu* (知熱灸) there either. I might do some other form of needling – you have seen this – or I might leave it altogether.

So I am looking for the idea of bringing the *Ki* inside. This is the 胃の気 (Stomach *Ki*). But remember that this is not simply the Stomach. It is the *Ki* you use for moving, activating – for being alive. For example, you can see it when looking at the pulse in the idea of a certain resilience or elasticity. Take a wiry pulse. If this resilient elastic quality is there then it shows a pulse with the ability to expand against an external pressure, but also to relax inwards. This is what I want to do with the abdominal needling. To allow the *Ki* (気) to relax inwards. But be sure to understand the difference between this relaxation and a state of collapse.

So in needling, I have the interaction of my own knowledge which is based on my experience and study - and the information I perceive by feeling and seeing right now.

TS: Does the same apply if we are doing the back *Shu* points (兪穴)?

EO: Ok – let me give you a piece of information which will help you a lot. In the beginning there were no points. In the beginning there were no meridians. So – how did they find it?

TS: Feeling...

EO: Yes – and by seeing. And then they put a name to it. Why did they do this?

TS: To help – to be able to pass it on?

EO: No.

TS: To remember it?

EO: Yes, could be. But even before that, in order to describe the effect – the phenomenon. So that found for example that this place affected the Liver energy so they called it *Kan Yu* (肝俞)。   They found that someone suffering from respiratory problems was helped by working here, so they called it *Hai Yu* (肺俞)。   And so on. So what is this state of mind – of the person that does this?

TS: Experimentation.

SB: Awareness.

EO: This is interesting. TS - you say "experimentation" and SB – you say "awareness. This is because you (TS) are coming from your brain – and you (SB) are coming from your senses. Get to know each other. Exchange vital fluids or something...

But – you see where I am coming from? Their treatment was alive. There was something active happening.

Brain

EO: Now look at the current teaching in schools – with a book and a teacher who says 'do this or that'. It is some sort of monstrosity – it is some sort of strange ritual or ceremony going on. For example, they decide it is a Lung problem – so they will go for the Lung point at all costs – even if there is no reaction there or anything going on. So the treatment is dead – it is something that happened in the book. But it is not happening in front of you.

Feeling

EO: Ok – now we go to the other extreme where the person decides he is just going to use his awareness. Here we have someone who hasn't learnt anything – it's all in what they feel. But then you have to ask yourself "what is the level of the person who is feeling? Can we train feeling?" You have to have some parameters within which to trust your feelings. And when you trust them you can develop them more – Or we can say 'uncover them more'. That comes from studying the theory. Then you get confidence enough to actually feel. And, not only that – you get the benefit of other people who have felt over the ages. And you can use it say – like floats in the water. Until you throw them away and you swim yourself. So it's ok to start like this. But don't confuse the start with the destination. You see – this is where the problem is.

2.3   ANTENNAE

EO: Don't tap the needle. And don't twist the needle either. Now, where is your intention/concentration?

MD: With the needle.

EO: Good. The arms are just here for decoration. They are just needed to complete the circuit/the ring. If you want to go a little deeper, just add pressure with the left fingers. Now, breathe. …From your arms to your wrists to your *Ro Kyu* (劳宫; PC8).

Patient[18]: Ow!

EO: Now, remember that. That is no good. This is a *Yang* deficient patient. For this point your hands and the needle are creating a mix. At the moment the needle part of the mix is too much. So, use your fingers a bit more to reduce the effect of the needle in the mix.

The needle is just a tool. The universe is passing through her body, the fingers and to the patient. That's the main thing here. If you use a needle, then the effect is stronger. Even if she just does a massage, the energy will reach the patient as long as it passes through her. However, with the needle, there's a greater effect.

We can think of acupuncturists, perhaps, as just antennas. Instead of rigid antennas, relaxed ones are more receptive. By including our intention, we greatly increase the absorption and release of this universe's energy.

In the case of a retained needle, this is also an antenna. However, without my intention it won't be able to have an intention. One last thing is the patient. Without a needle… just sitting and talking to the patient, Inserting *Ki*, seated meditation with the patient…these things also increase the absorption of the universe's *Ki*.

Anyway, as long as we relax the patient, we help that flow. That way, things from outside enter easily and things can also leave the patient's body more easily. The interesting thing with acupuncture is, even without the slightest bit of specialist knowledge, as long as you needle the painful area, the reduction in pain will lead to relief. This relief helps them relax. By relaxing the patient, the flow within their bodies improves. That helps get rid of bad things and also helps absorb the good things from outside.

We have to become better antennas. That's all. In order that we pick up

---

[18] In this case the patient was TS, one of the assisting practitioners.

more, sense more, receive more, we have to become better antennas. By using force, our antennas will give bad data. The flow will be a one-way thing from you to the patient only. Let's redefine *"Oriental Medicine"* to mean just becoming better antennas. And to help the patient also to become a better antenna.

2.4 FINDING POINTS ON THE BACK; PRISONERS IN THE IVORY TOWER

MD: How do you find the points on the back? Or how should we find the points on the back as we can't do it your way...

EO: Well – my way isn't fixed. My way is the same as yours except I have been doing it for longer. My way is to look for the points. That's the way you look.

The way you look will change, but the looking is the same. In fact I try just as hard if no harder than you do. And when I say look – this does not just mean with your eyes. It means your hands, your feeling – everything.

MD: So when you are doing the contact needling you are already examining where the deficiencies are – and you know where you want to go?

EO: Yes - I get a clearer idea. Also I prepare the body by increasing the *Ki* circulation so that the dents and the bumps become more exaggerated. If it is all tight then it is difficult to know. The contact needling improves the flow and thus reveals the places which remain hard and those which are relaxed. [EO gives an example of trying to find soft and hard areas on his contracted bicep and comparing that with the same search on a relaxed bicep]. It is the same as this but on a more subtle level. But the way to do it is to try and feel as much as you can. This doesn't change whether you have been doing it for one day or one year – 10 years. I am always trying to feel more – a better quality of perception. This remains the same but obviously you get better with practice. That's it.

The most important thing is never to leave your mind here [the head]. This is the worst place to have your mind. Put it outside of yourself – or in your hands – or through the patient – or through the needle. But whatever you do, never leave it in its box up here…you will be in trouble.

TS: It's taking a loooooong time, but I'm finally beginning to accept that this may actually be true.

EO: Actually it's not such a long time, TS. Some people never are able to see this.

TS: It doesn't mean that when you leave the clinic and want to study and look at the theory that you shouldn't go that way?

EO: Yes – but you need to understand this – people take that as "normal". The reality is that in the scheme of nature – that is for special occasions. For instance if a friend comes to you and is in trouble, the first thing is to go out of yourself and put yourself in his position. If you are in a dangerous position and you have a split second to decide you can't do it up here [in the head] – you have to just move. So actually having the mind in its ivory tower – you need to think of this as an unusual situation – not the norm. This is what I am trying to get over to you. You need to understand the difference between being a "prisoner" in there and a "visitor". You visit there with experiences from the outside which you can compare with the reference library up there. If you haven't been outside then you are in there as a prisoner. Everything you read and study in there is purely academic. So in order to make use of that material you have to go outside and experience it. Then you can digest and formulate. And then again you must come outside and test it.. This is constantly an in and out process. *Yin* and *Yang*. *Yin* and *Yang*.

But most people don't like it so much out there – they want to stay inside. You remember one of my patients was talking about his friend who wants to get married to a 2D manga character....

2.5   HANDS FOR NEEDLING

EO: Ok, your technique isn't too bad.

TS: So... ....what do I need to focus on?

EO: Your left hand – it has to relax – and pause - and actually become part of the patient – it is no longer you – it is the patient. Have a look at my left hand when I am needling - it is relaxed – in contact with the person. Your hands still need to develop to get this. *Ikeda Sensei* described it to me once – his hands changed and he said that he suddenly felt like a layer of plastic had been removed from between him and the patient – he could really feel. I'll tell you what I used to do – I used to practice for an hour – touch needling, one handed loading... then the technique becomes background – your hands change – become fuller.

2.6   KIDNEY MERIDIAN AND TONIFICATION

It is quite common in strong Kidney deficiency that the left meridian becomes tight – so I have to loosen it up before tonifying (eg at KI7). Otherwise I just end up tonifying the point and not the meridian. Now the process of needling is simply bringing my right hand toward my left – with the needle between. (The left hand is no longer mine – it is part of his body.) That creates an energy circuit.   If the left hand is not one with his body, all you feel is something after it happens.

2.7 NEEDLING *TAI KEI (KI3)*: *YIN-YANG* & THE IMPORTANCE OF HANDS

MD: When I'm needling *Tai Kei* (太谿; KI3), I don't feel comfortable with my 押し手 (*Oshide*)[19].

EO: It should be needled lightly so the 押し手 will be slightly different from normal. Let's have a look.

Wait! What is your purpose when needling that point? That must be made clear.

MD: I want to tonify the *Yin*.

EO: Oh, so you want to go into the *Yin* by going via 太谿 (*Tai Kei*; KI3)? Is that sound? 太谿 and *Yin* are actually contradicting each other. 太谿 is the Kidney's source point. Do we usually use source points to tonify the *Yin*? Usually, we use it for *Yang* deficiency. When you say *Yin*, what do you mean? *Yin* meridians?

MD: I mean the Blood.

EO: Also, if you are going to needle a little deeper on this point, then how deep is 'deep'? I'll show you one way. *Takenouchi Sensei* showed me how to do this and I used it for a number of years. The needle depth is a little less than 1cm and pulsing. This method is quite effective.

Now, let's think about MD's 押し手 why does it prick. How is it different?

MD: For *Yang* deficiency and 太谿 we don't needle deep. So, I try to softly needle and tonify the *Yang*. But, when I sometimes do it and

---

[19] 押し手 – This character is literally translated as the "the pushing/ holding hand". In refers to the position/ shape of the non-needling hand (usually the left).

the patient says it pricks, then I think that my 押し手 wasn`t steady enough..

EO: It isn`t a question of strength. Where`s the problem? Well, you don`t pierce the skin, first of all. Also, your hands... ...I think your hands need improving. Unfortunately, your hands don`t lie. Even *Ikeda Sensei*, when he gets tired, his hands get a little cold. When I get excited, my hands get a little sweaty. There are lots of reasons... ...like when you catch a cold. Anyway, the base of the base is good hands. Unfortunately, just improving the state of your hands is not possible, you have to do the whole body. Unless your whole body is *genki*[20], your hands won`t be either.

One more thing is, with *Yang* deficiency, you don`t fix the 押し手 too rigidly. If it`s too rigid, then you won`t register if you are pricking the skin or not.

The more you use strength, the less you will feel. But the other extreme - a wet sock - is also no good. A `waaaarrrrm` feeling being transmitted from your hand all the way to the far depths of the patient`s body is the best way. Don`t forget the feeling. That way, you will be able to register that the needle is pricking the skin.

2.8   NECK NEEDLING AND *DE CHI*

GW: Are we after *De Chi*?

EO: We aren`t actually after any of those things. We want to promote the flow of *Ki* and blood through that area. We know that if it's really tight, then it isn`t going to happen. And we know that if it's really loose, it isn't going to happen.

The areas that are really loose, we want to give a healthy tonus and get

---

[20] Japanese term meaning something like "in good, vibrant health".

the *Ki* and blood through there. The areas that are really tight, we want to loosen off and let the *Ki* and blood go through there nicely instead of being restricted. Now, in some cases there may be *De Chi* as a phenomena. In some cases they may say "気が至る" (the arrival of *Ki*). That may happen…OK?

GW: It's the same phenomena anyway, isn't it?

EO: It's not. It's different. *De Chi* is very physical.. it's just electricity-like. Whereas 至気 (arrival of *Ki*) is a little more subtle.

GW: Like the meridian getting a little warmer…?

EO: Yes like a pulsing beginning. Whereas the *De Chi*. I could do that before I went into school even… You just bung a needle in and boom. You know, that in itself is not consistent in bringing clinical results. Sometimes it is, but not always.. I've tried it, believe me.

GW: Is *De Chi* shunting?

EO: I guess it could be… …well, it's a phenomena..

GW: Oh, so it's just something separate…

EO: Yes - it could cause something. But then, on the other hand, it could cause nothing. It's like, "Is heat a phenomena of speed?" If I'm running very fast, then heat may be produced, but if I have a low wind resistance then the same speed may produce no heat. So, it's just one of the phenomena which we are focused on…

So we have to be careful to separate the phenomena. When you use a huge, thick needles exclusively, which some less-well trained practitioners do, then there is the danger that they just want to make sure they get it roughly in the area they need, which is a very tight, congested area. It's not very high level. But we know that it won't work in weak or deficient areas or patients. With that thin lady yesterday… …if you came in and used that approach of *De Chi* with her, what result would you have?

2.9   NEEDLING THE NECK (& *WU WEI*)

EO: One thing is that the choice of where I go and you go is different. So I go where I can go in. You are trying to go through a brick wall whereas I am using the door. Here it is, it must go in.

TS: Ok – so if I find it's not going in…

EO: Leave it. Because for you at that time to do it is not right – it might be your level – or the choice of point. Or perhaps it's just the patient. Anyway – at that time it's not right.

TS: Yes – at some times it just goes in – with no problem.

EO: OK – then that is the correct time to use it. Look, if there is resistance then he is creating it. It's not just here – it's all over the body. This resistance will of course have a negative effect on the treatment. Remember – it will have an effect over the whole body. You are not doing this needling just for the area. Also you must make sure that you are not just trying to get him to do something which actually you want him to do – which is not at his pace. It's like a consensus. You have to listen to see if the consensus is really in place or not. Like a conversation – you have to get agreement. You don't just go in there unilaterally. Otherwise you can get a short term response but its unlikely to lead to any deep healing. Of course we can't just leave him here on the couch and ask him to pay on the way out. He won't get much better. But if I simply impose my ideas about how he is going to get better and if he is ready or not… we don't want that either. You can feel all of that actually going on with the needle. If there is resistance then you can spend a little bit of time until they let go. But if they don't then you go somewhere else. Leave it. It means that door isn't open at that time for you. This means one of two things. Either you haven't got the key ("*Ki*") for that door. Or it means that door is not really there.

And you are banging your head against a brick wall.

...*Wu Wei*...

This is what they mean when they talk of *Wu Wei* (無為). This does not actually mean "doing nothing" – it means rather doing nothing that is unnecessary. So if he is tensing up and I am forcing my way through it then I am doing the wrong thing. I am not acting in accordance with *Wu Wei*. But if I take it here and the body relaxes and is open then it's ok. It's appropriate. Also I haven't got in my mind the idea about doing something and using the profit motive – thinking ahead and predicting the result. No. So it leaves you much more free and natural. And stronger, actually. Because he gets ready and when he's ready then I can help him.

TS:　　　Yes – I realised that I was also tight when I was trying to needle him.

EO:　　　Yes – so if you are tight – this is also on a deeper and more subtle level – then it must transfer to him. It must because he is completely defenseless, lying there, opening himself up to you needling him. So anything that you do goes in deeper. So then you have to just go with what is in front of you.

2.10　Shunting

CH:　　　I have a question – someone gets a cold or some acute symptom and then they get *Kan Jitsu* (肝実; Liver Excess)....like *Hai Kyo Kan Jitsu* (肺虚肝実; Lung deficiency Liver excess). Does this pulse look different from a chronic case of *Kan Jitsu*?

EO:　　　Yes. Because one is blood stagnation and the other is heat.

CH:　　　Ok - when you use *Ko Kan* (LV2) - is this taking out the heat by increasing the fluids (as it's the fire point) or is its action by releasing the whole meridian?

EO: It's both. One is by increasing the fluids – cooling it. The other way – is because I am doing it against the flow of the meridian I am stopping the centripetal flow of the meridian. Not stopping it completely but easing it…

TS: Ok – if you are going deep and shunting to increase the fluids…we can think of this as a tonification of the *Yin*. If this is the case, why is going against the flow of the meridian tonification?

EO: Well, it's not tonification, it's shunting. I think you are not clear on the use of the term. At one specific moment we have a number of choices to make and we are using our sensitivity – and we need extreme flexibility at that moment in time. This means that the basics must be very clearly defined. Because you are going to use these tools to be flexible. If those basic principles are not very clearly defined and you then wish to be flexible on top of that shakey foundation…then….

So you have to be careful about the terms you want to use. Do it now so we can get to the root of your confusion. So, when we use *Ko Kan* (LV2), we are ending up with a net result of what we call shunting. Define shunting.

TS: Well – one way is to think of it as tonifying the *Yin* of that meridian. Because we are going deep – and we are trying to move – or shunt – something from one place to another.

EO: Alright – then we are getting a mix there. Tonifying the *Yin* of the meridian will have a new result of cooling. But the shunting will have the result of taking one thing from one place to another – from where it is not needled to where it is.

TS: Ok – the way I put those two things together is that if you are shunting there must be an excess (local at least) there – otherwise why shunt… So an excess is a build-up which results in heat and therefore by tonifying the *Yin*, you cool the area and the flow improves resulting in the shunting from that place of excess. So – if this reasoning is acceptable, then why do I want to go against the flow – I am tonifying (*Yin*) and I want the flow to go in the direction of nature to move.

EO: What it means is this. The Liver Meridian is moving inwards and making the blood gather here more than it should. So we can cool the meridian by tonifying the *Yin*. Which by definition means that we can say it is being shunted – in this we are in agreement. At the same I can come in against the flow to impede the gathering a little. So I can get a lot of effect for less than usual effort. With both of these actions.

TS: I have been through this thought process but I can also see an alternative argument....the way that I...

EO: Hold on – now this is just like changing hats... ...do you like me in this one or that one... This is important. Because if you do this you want arrive at a principle. You will end up with a number of ways of looking at it, none of which will amount to a principle.

TS: I understand the point you are making. But...

EO: I want you to be careful – because you have an active brain, but I want it to engage in principles.

TS: Ok – the principle that I have arrived at is this: When I want to shunt, I want to cool things down so as to improve the flow of the meridian.

EO: But if the flow of the meridian is moving inwards and you improve the flow then it will gather even more...

TS: Except that because I am tonifying the *Yin* of the Meridian – this is the principle if you like – what I am tonifying is the cooling aspect. I am re-populating the fluids in the meridian and the organ rather than gathering the blood.

CH: That's more like *Kan Kyo In Kyo* (Liver Deficiency *Yin*

Deficiency)…

EO: Yes – that would be better for *Kan Kyo In Kyo* (Liver Deficiency *Yin* Deficiency).

TS: But you seem to have a different principle for that.

EO: No no – it's the same principle. You could use that on the GB meridian where there is a lot of heat and you would come in and tonify the *Yin*.

TS: Yes – but it would be in the direction of the meridian…

EO: Yes – yes you can do that.

TS: So why is there a different principle for *In Kyo* (*Yin* Deficiency) and *Kan Jitsu* (Liver excess)?

EO: Well – it is a different state – one is deficient heat, one is excess heat. But think about it in these terms: You can come in like that and it will have a reasonable effect. What you will do is you will still have blood gathering in the Liver but there will be more fluids. But if possible you want to reduce the gathering. Because at that time it is stealing from somewhere else. That's why we call it shunting – because if possible we want to stop the gathering (stealing) so that another organ – the Kidney in most cases – can keep some of its fluids.

2.11 BURNING QUESTIONS

Q   Meridian- therapy seems to use tonification in the treatment of every type of pattern, whether excess or deficient. Colds are classified as external excess conditions. Why is it appropriate to tonify in this condition?

The *Wei Jing* (内経; Internal Classic) states that: "*All disease arises from a deficiency of the Yin organs.*" In the case of a cold, the Lungs are usually too weak to circulate defensive *Ki* properly, allowing pathogenic *Ki* to enter the body via the *Yang* meridians. Thus tonifying the Lung will strengthen the circulation of defensive *Ki* to allow the body to dispel the pathogen.

While it is always necessary to tonify the deficient *Yin* meridian(s), dispersion of *Yang* meridians may also be required. This is the case if an excess is detected in the *Yang* meridians when taking the pulse after tonifying the *Yin* meridians

It should also be noted that I do not necessarily represent meridian therapy, but aim to advance the practice of acupuncture and moxibustion through the use of ideas and techniques which have been found to be consistently effective in the clinic. In particular, referring regularly to the classics for the foundation of practice and endeavouring to maintain a flexible approach at all times is recommended. This flexibility ensures that the options available for approaches to treatment are never exhausted.

Q   Does Japanese acupuncture always use shallow needling with thin needles? How would a Japanese acupuncturist treat cases of bi syndrome, in which there is pain deep in the joints or the muscles are extremely stiff?

First, it is impossible to define Japanese acupuncture. It has been estimated that in Japan only 20% of practitioners in Japan use traditional forms of diagnosis, e.g. pulse and tongue examination, when practising acupuncture.

Practitioners using techniques similar to those used by *Ikeda Sensei* are in a very small minority. Generally, it is true to say that thinner needles are used in Japanese acupuncture; however, the number of Japanese practitioners utilizing specialized techniques such as using the *Shin Kan* (鍼管; guide tube) as a tonification or dispersion tool is relatively small. As a rule, we use shallow (to a depth of 1 mm) or contact needling when tonifying. Stiff, painful, or tight areas needled to a depth of 2—3 mm, into what is referred to as the nutritive *Ki* level.

Although shallow needling is used most commonly, it is often necessary to needle more deeply, i.e. to a depth of 1—2 cm, and sometimes to use Chinese needles. However, this type of needling is considered to be strong stimulation and is never used on patients showing signs of *Yang* deficiency, i.e. those who have a deep, thin or weak pulse. Deep needling can safely be used on patients with evident blood stagnation or relatively strong deficient heat. Areas that have been very stiff or tight on a long-term basis are the best candidates for deep needling.

The site to be needled should be selected very carefully by palpating to find a depres-sion within the hard or stiff area. The left hand is used to prepare the point by kneading and pressing, opening up the point. Care must be taken not to needle more points than is necessary.

Note also that moxa is extensively used together with needling because it would be more difficult to get the desired results with needling alone. Thus a patient with joint or muscle pain would always be treated using a type(s) of moxibustion. Moxa has the advantage of being able to penetrate deep into tight areas to relax them without causing the discomfort associated with strong dispersive needling.

2.12 WHAT IS THE NEEDLE?

Sometimes a patient would say something like "鍼は良く効くね。。。 (*acupuncture is very effective, isn't it....*)". And I remember once *Takenouchi Sensei* putting a needle onto the bed in-front of the patient and saying "Ok - are you feeling any better now?". Obviously the patient would responded that there was no effect and *Takenouchi Sensei* would say something like "Ok - well it's not just the needle, is it?"

I don't know for sure what he meant by saying this because he was very old and I was very young and there was therefore immediately a gap between our views on the world. But I took from it what a young man should learn at that time. But one thing we can say is that although we talk about needles and that we are inserting here and there... ...actually the biggest aerial is not the needle - it is us! Look at the size of us compared to the needle.

This piece of wire is simply something that concentrates it. It has no inherent power to heal.

So the more we can get this totality of ourselves clear and able to act as an antennae then of course the needle is able to be imbued with some healing effect.

Most of the time we concentrate so much on the needle that we miss the most important thing. Which is actually everything else but the needle. How is the patient feeling? How is their flow of *Ki*? How are their tissues? How are they changing? How is the skin underneath the needle feeling? That is why they talk about the left hand so much. It has the meaning not just of the importance of the left hand - but of everything else *apart* from the needle. This is how I am thinking about it...

So do we need the needle? How about we *become* the needle? We leave our intentions behind and then techniques flow and ebb and are born in an instant to fit the unique circumstance in front of us - and real healing can take place.

We have to be careful - because the needle has its place. It doesn't lead us - we lead it.

2.13 HAND CRAFTED NEEDLES[21]

There is an old English saying which goes, "*A bad craftsman always blames his tools*." In the case of the acupuncturist the "tools of the trade" are his needles and many times they are blamed for the difficulties which occur during treatment. Even though these often criticized needles are used countless times by acupuncturists, it is surprising how little the average practitioner knows about his tools. In an effort to rectify this situation, the following article was written in the belief that: "*A good craftsman knows and respects his tools*".

NEEDLE CRAFTSMAN

It was my great pleasure and privilege to meet *Kinichi Aoki* and his son *Tsuneo* at his needle-workshop in *Mejiro*, Japan, and it was from Mr. *Aoki* that a valuable insight into the art of needling was obtained. Mr. *Aoki* is a quiet, dignified 74 year old man who represents the third generation of needle makers in the *Aoki* family. The needle-making tradition was started by Mr. *Aoki* 's grandfather, a practising acupuncturist who was not satisfied with the needles available at that time and decided to make his own.

From the time that Mr. *Aoki* 's grandfather was alive until quite recently the needle maker was considered to be socially superior to the acupuncturists who used his needles. Thus it was with great care that Mr. *Aoki* 's grandfather and father selected suitable acupuncturists who were then able to purchase their needles. Nowadays of course, Mr. *Aoki* recognises that he has to earn a living but since the demand for his needles far exceeds his production he still maintains an element of selection in his clients.

---

[21] This Article was first printed in the British Journal of Acupuncture 10:1 1987, before the Author had enrolled in Acupuncture college in Tokyo.

For Mr. *Aoki* (and his son) needle-making is not merely a livelihood but an art and a service to the sick. Each batch of needles therefore is special, but Mr. *Aoki* has one particular batch that he is most proud of. This is the batch made for Dr. *Inoue* who heads a clinic located in *Ikebukuro* in Tokyo. Dr. *Inoue* uses his own individual acupuncture techniques (light, quick, shallow, piercing of the skin) and thus required his own custom-made needles composed of a longer than average needle head and a shorter, thinner needle shaft. Mr. *Aoki* very much enjoyed crafting such a needle and was very happy when the finished product met with Dr. *Inoue's* approval, who, incidentally, had previously tried other needle makers and had not gained any satisfaction.

Mr. *Aoki* 's hands betray their trade by the unusual length of the nails of his thumb and little finger which is necessary in order to pick up the very fine gauge of needles which he makes. Needle-making, however, is not the only skill which his hands possess; he also is a very keen photographer. Indeed his photography is excellent as is evidenced by the framed photographs that can be seen displayed at his workshop. In his youth he won a very prestigious photography prize which resulted in a lot of publicity including an article about him in the newspaper. This was, as he recalls, quite fine but as he humourously remarked it had one drawback. After discovering the article about this "young, virile" photographer the army immediately drafted him. Photography requires a certain aesthetic, artistic sense and needle making requires precision and attention to detail. It is a combination of these qualities that is the hallmark of the *Aoki* needle: aesthetic and satisfying while being precise and well finished.

NEEDLE HEAD PRODUCTION

Firstly a block of 99% pure silver is rolled into a thin 0.25mm sheet (Figure 2-2-a). (All needle heads in Mr. *Aoki* 'sworkshop are made of silver regardless of whether the shaft is made of gold or silver).

The rolled sheet of silver is then cut into thin strips (Figure 2-2-b). At this stage one end of each strip is rounded to produce a curled tip. (Figure 2-2-c).

The strips are then passed through progressively smaller holes until a tube diameter of 1.3mm is obtained (Figure 2-2-d).

The narrow tubes are now partially cut by being rolled back and forth under the sharp edge of a heavy knife. They are then broken into sections representing the needle head. A copper section is then inserted into the silver tubes and filed down to size in preparation for soldering the needle-shaft to the head (Figure 2-2-e).

The resulting section composed of a thin silver tube and a copper core is the needle head which is now ready to be attached to the needle shaft.

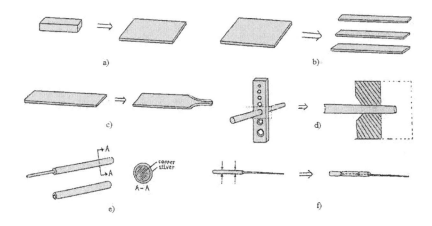

Figure 2-2: Needle Head & Shaft Production

Needle Head: a) Block of silver rolled into sheet; b) Sheet is cut into strips; c) One end of each strip is rounded; d) Rounded end is forced through holes to produce a narrow tube; e) Copper section inserted inside the tube. Needle Shaft: f) Needle shaft joined to needle head using solder method or press method.

NEEDLE SHAFT PRODUCTION

Gold and silver have always been favoured for the needle shaft as they are soft metals and cause less pain upon initial insertion. They are also chemically very stable (due to their atomic structure) and thus attract less bacteria.

Silver shafts are made from wires of a composition of 80% silver (Ag) and 20% copper (Cu) and zinc (Zn). Gold shafts are made from wires of 20 carat gold (pure gold is 24 carats), the remaining 4/24 consists of copper (Cu). The wires are pulled through progressively smaller holes to produce thin wires of the desired diameter. The process is similar to that carried out for the needle head production except that the scale is a lot smaller and that industrial diamonds are used to shape the wire diameter. Generally the needle shaft diameters are made to an accuracy of 1/100mm[22]. The resulting needles are as follows:

No. 3 Gauge needle = 0.197mm diameter[23]
No. 4 Gauge needle = 0.417mm diameter
No. 5 Gauge needle = 0.637mm diameter

The needle shafts are now cut to the required length using scissors and then joined to the needlehead.

JOINING NEEDLE SHAFT & HEAD

There are basically two methods of joining the needle shaft and head together: the "solder" method and the "pressed" method. Both have their advantages and disadvantages.

---

[22] This accuracy of 1/100 for hand-made needles cannot really be improved upon while using the process of progressively smaller holes to form the diameters. This is because with time the holes themselves become slightly worn (and thus expanded) due to the metal sections constantly being drawn through them.
[23] The difference in diameter between each Gauge is 0.22mm.

Solder Method

In this method the needle head is placed on pre-heated oak charcoal (*Kashi*). Solder is melted on to one end of the needle shaft which is then inserted into the softened end of the head. The solder method is the older of the two methods and has the advantage that it gives a very firm secure feeling when handling the needle with little or no wobble occuring. The two major disadvantages are (i) that because the needle shaft is fixed solidly into the needle head it tends to be inflexible which makes the joint more vulnerable to stress; and (ii) the soldered head is prone to melting, thereby causing the needles to become useless when sterilized in an autoclave.

Pressed method

With the increased stress placed on sterilization methods brought about by the concern over B-Type Hepatitis and more recently AIDS, the pressed joint needle, which can better withstand the high pressure of the autoclave, provides an alternative to the solder head needle. In this method the needle head contains no copper core. The needle head simply has the needle shaft inserted inside it and is pressed by a clamp which dents the head casing producing a vice-like grip on the needle shaft. Clamping usually starts from 1/3 of the length of the needle head from the joint thus allowing a certain amount of flexibility and reducing the stress at the joint. Note that for needles made using the press-method no copper core is inserted into the needle head tube.)

The number of clamps required increases in proportion to the slenderness in needle shaft diameter, i.e. a very thin needle shaft requires many clamps. Mechancially one disadvantage of the pressed needle head is that it tends to be over-mobile at the joint, giving a needle that tends to wobble easily and lack firmness. This same trait, however, gives rise to a benefit in that it reduces the stress at the joint, making breakage less likely to occur.

Generally among modern practitioners it appears that pressed needle head needles are more popular due to their wide use of autoclave sterilization.

SHAPING THE TIP OF THE NEEDLE HEAD

There are 4 needle tip shapes that are commonly used; they are *Surioroshin*, *Noge*, *Tamago* (Egg) and *Matsuba* (Pine needle) shaped. Mr. *Aoki* creates needles that are shaped mid-way between *Tamago* and *Matsuba* shaped needles. Shaping of the tip of the needle head is a four-fold process involving grinding the needle tip using successively finer grinders[24]. The first grinder uses a grinding head of stone. This is followed by a nylon-felt grinder, a woolen-felt grinder and finally a cotton-buffer grinder.

QUALITY CONTROL

Quality control in Mr. *Aoki* 's workshop is done on a random basis by means of a microscopic examination.

INSERTION TUBES

Nowadays, 90% of insertion tubes are of the hexagonal variety although originally they were round because of their origins in fashioned bamboo. An interesting background story concerning the hexagonal shape is that when acupuncture became the domain mainly of blind practitioners, They had many problems with round shaped tubes because when placed on a surface they would roll a long distance making it difficult, if not impossible, to find. The hexagonal shape could be put down in one place and not roll away. Hexagonal insertion tubes are not usually made from scratch by the needle workshop nowadays. Rather thay are obtained from the foundry in pre-rolled sections. At the workshop long metallic tubes are cut and polished to size.

---

[24] Using grinders of 2.000-3.000 rpm

In the past the insertion tubes were made from scratch, i.e. the metal was beaten into sheets which were then joined together and pounded into shape. Unfortunately the amount of labour involved was enormous and thus today it is rarely if ever done.

Many practitioners, regardless of the type of needle they use, prefer to use a gold or silver insertion tube.

One of the chief reasons is that gold and silver tubes are expensive and symbolise a pride in and commitment to one's profession which affects both the practitioner and patient psychologically. A simple analogy is that of a concert pianist. if he were to give a concert using a second-grade piano; it would not be a success. Even if he played and sounded perfect, he wouldn't feel comfortable and neither would the audience.

Another more subtle, yet I believe more valid reason for using gold and silver insertion tubes is to do with *Ki*. At Mr. *Aoki* 's workshops, I was able to touch and appreciate insertion tubes made of stainless steel, silver (of varying purities) and gold. Even to my relatively inexperienced grasp the conclusion to be reached was obvious. The stainless steel tube felt dead, cold and artificial. The gold and silver tubes on the other hand, felt alive and quickly warmed to the touch becoming "part of me" in a very short time. Simplistically speaking, gold and silver conduct heat more readily than stainless steel. Now *Ki* can be thought of as similar to heat or electrical energy of the body and it can be concluded that using silver or gold insertion tubes allows the practitioner to more easily transfer his *Ki* to the patient - an important part of any treatment programme.

CONCLUSION

After visiting Mr. *Aoki* 's workshop and talking with him and his son, needles were no longer just implements to be used - but real quality tools of the healing profession to be valued and appreciated. Fine wine is not to be gulped down but rather to be savoured and enjoyed with full knowledge of its heritage and characteristics. It is my hope that acupuncturists everywhere will learn to value their needles in the same way.

CHAPTER 3

Moxibustion (お灸; *Okyu*)

3.1 INTRODUCTION TO MOXIBUSTION

INTRODUCTION

Moxibustion is the therapeutic practice of burning moxa (艾; *mogusa*), a tinder made from the dried leaves of *Artemisia princeps* (*vulgaris*), commonly known as mugwort (蓬; *yomogi*), on or near the skin. The roots of heat therapy can be traced to the natural urge of people living in cold climates to warm up painful areas. Over time, they found various ways of transferring heat to the body, one of the first being stones heated to a suitable temperature pressed onto the skin.

One of the earliest references to moxibustion is in chapter 12 of the Simple Questions (素問) (*So Mon* in Japanese, *Su Wen* in Chinese), which deals with different treatment methods:

異法方宜論第十二篇
北方者，天地所閉藏之域也，其地高陵居，風寒冰
冽，其民樂野處而乳食，藏寒生滿病，其治宜灸
焫，故灸焫者，亦從北方來。

The north is the area where things are closed off in storage.
The mountains and the hills where the people dwell have
bitterly cold, icy winds. The tribes of this area lead a nomadic
existence, eating mainly dairy products. This causes the
people to have chilled internal organs, resulting in full
diseases. The most appropriate treatment for this is
moxibustion. Thus it can be seen that moxibustion originated
in the north.

The ideograms " 滿病" are used to describe "full diseases," which are characterized by swelling and fullness of the chest and Stomach. The large amount and widespread consumption of dairy products is now often cited in connection with a number of diseases. Therefore it is of value to examine what is meant by the term "full disease" mentioned in this 2000 year old text. The ideogram 滿 can be split as follows:

$$滿 = 氵 + 艹 + 入入$$
$$\quad\quad\; 1 \quad\quad 2 \quad\quad 3$$

1.   means water all over, all around;
2.   means left and right in perfect balance;
2 +3.   means a set of scales or a balance, level and completely full.

Therefore the whole character literally means a vase or pond full of water, which fills every nook and cranny. In this context, " 滿病" refers to diseases characterized by fullness in the chest and abdominal regions, including gas, bloating, Liver cirrhosis, tumours, both benign and malignant, and the final stages of cancer, characterized by hydropsis.

Commentators examining the above passage of the *So Mon* tend to focus on the origin of moxibustion in the north, but the passage also tells us the following:

1. Environmental factors and dairy products may cause chilling of the internal organs;

2. Chilling of the internal organs causes "full" diseases such as abdominal and chest distension, Liver cirrhosis, and tumours of various types; and

3. These full diseases are best treated using moxibustion.

Tumors often produce abnormally high body temperatures, and frequently, when palpated locally in areas such as the abdomen, they are warmer than the surrounding areas. This is due to the body desperately trying to supply the growing tumour with nourishment. It is almost as if the body has tried to correct the chilling by creating heat, but is unable to do so smoothly and uniformly, resulting in the formation of heat lumps (tumours).

Recently in Japan stomach cancer and viral infection have been linked. When the body is run down and the internal temperature drops slightly, the bacterial-viral balance of the body is altered, allowing immune system dysfunction and thus disease. In the West, particularly where there has always been a large intake of dairy products, diseases such as cancer have claimed many lives.

This and the implications of the passage from *So Mon* suggest that moxibustion may prevent chilling of the internal organs and thus ultimately both benign and malignant tumours. For this reason, in Japan, moxibustion, particularly loquat leaf moxibustion, is used to combat cancer. Of course, changing the diet is also important, with particular attention on the effect of dairy products and other chilling factors on the body [25]. From the perspective of the immune system, regular moxibustion has wide- ranging positive results which is a prerequisite for health and prevention of disease.

WHAT IS MOXIBUSTION

Moxibustion is the application of thermal stimulation to specific areas of the body to restore balanced function. It consists of burning processed yomogi leaves either directly or indirectly on the skin. Before explaining the basic techniques used in moxibustion, I would like to outline the constituents and production of moxa.

Constituents of Moxa

Moxa formed from *yomogi* has the following constituents:

1.   Water;

2.   Protein;

3.   Carbohydrate;

4.   Essential oils, including cineole, thujone, sesquiterpene, etc;

5.   Fats, including palmitic acid, oleic acid, linolenic acid, and stearic acid;

6.   Wax, including cerotic acid and ceryl alcohol;

7.   Enzymes such as amylase, catalase, ascorbic acid, and invertin; and

8.   Vitamins A, B1, B2, C, etc

---

[25] This is not meant to suggest that all dairy products are harmful to health; yoghurt for instance is an excellent food. Excessive, inappropriate use of dairy products is referred to here. For more details, please refer to explanations of macrobiotic theory, such as those by *Michio Kushi* and George *Ohsawa*.

Production of moxa

Yomogi is harvested, normally in May or June, dried, and ground into a fluffy soft material -moxa. Certain areas in China and Japan are known for moxa production; in China, *Honanshen* is one such area. In Japan, moxa produced in Ibukiyama is considered to be of the highest quality. However, currently *Niigata, Toyama,* and *Nagano* prefectures are among the main growing areas, with *Niigata* now being responsible for 80% of the moxa production in Japan.

The typical production process is as follows:

1. *Yomogi* leaves are harvested between May and the beginning of August;

2. The leaves are dried in natural sunlight for 5 days by the farmers;

3. At the end of August, the dried yomogi is collected from the farmers and stored at a moxa factory;

4. Around the end of November, when the weather begins to get very cold, moxa production proper begins;

5. The moxa to be prepared for the following day is put into a charcoal-heated drying room for one day;

6. The moxa is then put into a grinding mill (in many cases this is still done by hand), the rough ground product being suitable for warming moxibustion;

7. Depending on the desired quality of the moxa, the grinding is repeated;

8. Green particles, stems, etc are removed;

9. The remaining portion is put into a *Tomi* (唐箕), a tumbler/fanning machine, where the moxa receives its final treatment, which removes any fine particles and produces a fluffy consistency.

Quality

The quality of moxa can be judged using the information provided in Table 3-1.

Moxa Quality	Good Quality	Poor Quality
Smell	Old, Good smell	New, Raw smell
Fell	Soft, Thin Fibers	Hard, Thick fibers
Colour	Pale yellow	Darkish green
Purity	Few impurities	Many impurities
Moisture	Dry, Fluffy	Damp, Lumpy
Burning	Leaves little ash	Leaves much ash
Burning	Easily ignited	Difficult to ignite
Burning	Little smoke	Much smoke
Heat	Soft, Pleasant	Harsh, Unbearable

Table 3-1: Comparison of Moxa Quality

MOXIBUSTION TECHNIQUES

There are two basic methods of applying moxibustion:

1. Scarring moxibustion, which utilizes a third-degree burn to achieve therapeutic results; and

2. Non-scarring moxibustion, which utilizes a first or second-degree burn to achieve therapeutic results.

*1. Scarring moxibustion (*有痕灸*; Yu Kon Kyu)*

Scarring moxibustion is the application of moxibustion directly to the skin, producing a scar of varying, although usually small, size. The quality of the moxa used is better than that used for non-scarring moxibustion. Practitioners of direct moxibustion (at least in Japan) endeavour to give an effective treatment but also to ensure that the scar is as small and neat as possible, if not actually beautiful. Scars that last are often a matter of pride for the patient and also display the handiwork of the practitioner; therefore tremendous skill and care go into making each cone.

This is one of the main reasons why this technique is not so popular with the average practitioner: it is difficult to perform and therefore easier to omit, excuses such as, *"The patients don't like it"* or the old favourite, *"It doesn't feel right"* being cited. These people are absolutely correct; something insufficiently practised and poorly executed will feel wrong to the practitioner and will be detested by the patient! However, scarring moxibustion is without doubt the most powerful tool available to the acupuncturist and deserves serious study and great effort.

Penetrating moxibustion (透熱灸; *To Netsu Kyu*)

Penetrating moxibustion is the method most widely practised in Japan and involves burning small (rice grain- or half rice grain-sized) cones of moxa on selected points on the skin. This method is used to drill heat into the skin and is similar to a hot needle, penetrating deep into the body. Penetrating moxibustion is used mostly to tonify, but can also be used for dispersion.

Cautery moxibustion (焦灼灸; *Sho Shaku Kyu*)

Cautery moxibustion is used to destroy unwanted tissue such as verrucas, warts, and corns. In this technique, tightly rolled, reasonable large (rice-grain size or larger) moxa cones are burnt repeatedly directly on affected areas. Ten treatments at once- or twice-weekly intervals are normally enough to clear up even the most stubborn cases, and the recurrence rate is very low.[26]

---

[26] The author has obtained good results with this method, even in cases where laser and dry ice treatments have failed. Recurrence was not observed over a 3-year follow-up period.

Suppurative moxibustion (打膿灸; *Da No Kyu*)

Suppurative moxibustion is currently not often used, but involves deliberately creating a limited suppurative or festering area. Utilizing the body's response to this process, chronic diseases can be overcome and greater resistance is generally produced..

The suppuration is achieved by burning between one and three thumb-sized cones of moxa directly on the skin, leaving a large burn. A resinous cream is then applied to the burn to encourage the suppurative process. The cream is administered and the burn dressed with gauze every day for 40 to 50 days until it is healed, the scar resulting from this process was traditionally described as being like "the eye of the horse." However, before the widespread use of antibiotics it served as a last resort means for dealing with chronic diseases.[27]

2. Non-scarring moxibustion (無痕灸; Mu Kon Kyu)

Indirect moxibustion (隔物灸; *Kaku Butsu Kyu*)

Indirect moxibustion is a form of moxibustion in which a substance is placed between the burning moxa and the skin. The substance reduces the heat of the moxa and is transferred into the body via the skin. The moxa used in this technique is of a lower grade than that used for scarring moxibustion. Many substances can be placed between the skin and the moxa; some of the more common are as follows:

1. Garlic (大蒜; *Niniku*) is used to improve blood circulation and generally warm up the body;

2. *Miso* (味噌), which is derived from soya beans, is good for the Stomach and Spleen and ensures that heat is distributed evenly;

---

[27] In my clinical practice, elderly patients (70 years) sometimes display signs of *Da No Kyu*, normally around the upper back. Further investigation reveals that the technique was used mostly for pneumonia, tuberculosis, and other upper respiratory tract disorders.

3. Ginger (生姜; *Shoga*) is also used to warm the body and is especially favoured for use in female sterility and difficulty in conception;

4. Salt (塩; *Shio*) is found in almost any house-hold, spreads moxa heat uniformly, and is used traditionally for gastrointestinal problems, particularly diarrhoea;

5. Loquat leaf (枇杷; *Biwa*) boosts the immune system by cleansing the blood, and is used for serious illnesses including cancer (one of its active ingredients is known to be vitamin B17, a constituent of natural anticancer drugs); and

6. Last but not least is moxa, which drives all the other substances into the body and is derived from yomogi, which has been used as a health tonic, an antifebrile, diuretic, antihelmintic, hemostatic, and antiseptic agent, a gastrointestinal stimulant, etc. in Japan for centuries.

7. Loquat leaf is of particular interest because it has disappeared from use in China and Korea. The origins of loquat leaf can be traced to the Buddha, who is said to have used the leaves of the Loquat to help the sick 2500 years ago. In the sutras, the loquat tree is referred to as the "king medicinal tree" and the leaves as "fans to relieve distress" due to their shape and medicinal properties. With the spread of Buddhism, loquat leaf therapy entered China, where it was eventually combined with acupuncture and herbal medicine. From China via Korea, loquat was introduced into Japan about 1500 years ago (during the *Nara* Period), where it has been developed almost exclusively in Buddhist temples up to the present.

Although introduced from China and Korea, loquat leaf is no longer used in these countries and therefore it is to Japan that loquat leaf therapy owes its modern development. Traditionally loquat leaves were pressed onto the skin using a lighted moxa stick with some damp gauze or similar material in between. The extract of the leaf was transferred by heat and pressure onto the skin. Nowadays more convenient and effective methods are available, whereby an extract of the leaf in an alcohol base is steamed onto the skin using moxa heat.

During trips to Korea, Taiwan, and China, I have enquired as to the use of loquat in traditional medicine, but have discovered that it appears to be used only in herbal remedies, mainly for the throat.

However, in Japan, in addition to its use herbally, there are societies that specialize in loquat leaf moxibustion, and it is used in some hospitals for incurable diseases.

Warming moxibustion (温灸; *On Kyu*)

As the name suggests, in warming moxibustion, moxa or a device of some kind is used to warm the area or point.

1. **Stick moxibustion** *(棒灸; Bo Kyu).* In stick moxibustion, a rolled stick of moxa is used to warm the skin. If used properly it can restore balance to the entire body and is one of the simplest but most often used form of moxibustion in Chinese acupuncture.

2. **Heat perception moxibustion** (知熱灸; *Chi Netsu Kyu*). This technique employs a large cone of moxa placed directly on the skin. The cone is lit and allowed to burn until the patient perceives first a pleasant warmth and then more intense heat. At this time a signal is given and the cone is swiftly removed. This method is believed to have originated in Japan and is a mainstay of those practising the "meridian therapy" style of acupuncture. Heat perception moxibustion is very effective when used on the stomach and shoulders, and is normally attached to the skin using a small dab of

Shi Un Ko[28]. *Chi Netsu Kyu* is very relaxing and pleasurable, and leaves a gentle warmth that patients love.

3. ***Platform moxibustion*** *(台灸; Dai Kyu)* is the mounting of moxa above the skin to leave a small air pocket between the burning moxa and the skin. This allows warmth to be imparted without burning the skin. In this technique, the moxa heat is adjusted carefully so as to hover between a first and second degree burn. Inferior types of platform moxibustion often cross the line and result in a blister burn worse than the burn that would result if direct scarring moxibustion were to be applied. A good example of this type of moxibustion is Kamaya Mini Kyu (weak [green] version), which enjoys considerable popularity in Japan.

4. ***Needle head moxibustion*** *(灸頭鍼; Kyu To Shin)* is the application of moxa heat deep into the tissues through acupuncture needles. A ball of moxa is placed on the head of a reasonably deeply inserted needle and lit. The penetration of heat into the tissues results in deep tonification of *Yin*. This technique is frequently used for chronic conditions and is also believed to have originated in Japan.

5. ***Needle shaft moxibistion*** *(灸根鍼; Kyu Kon Shin)* is similar to *Kyu To Shin*, but stick moxa is used to heat the shaft of the needle. This method appears to have been developed by *Misao Takenouchi*, and can be used for both deep and shallow tonification.

6. ***Device moxibustion*** *(機械灸; Ki Kai Kyu)* uses various devices, electrical or otherwise, to impart warmth to the skin. A good example of this is the infrared lamp used by many practitioners from various disciplines.

---

[28]紫雲膏. Literally translated these characters mean "purple cloud ointment." This ointment is used for all types of skin disorders, including burns, and is a Japanese formulation.

EFFECTS OF MOXIBUSTION

The effects of moxibustion on the organism have been researched in Japan since the early 1900s; however, most of the data available, although valuable, are unfortunately from the first half of this century. Research started due to the pressure under which oriental medicine was placed by the reforms introduced by the Meiji government (1868-1912). In later years these data were to be extremely useful in resisting pressure from the occupation forces, led by General MacArthur, who nearly destroyed the practice of moxibustion by banning its use completely, believing it to be an instrument of torture. It was only after experiments proving that moxibustion is therapeutic were re-examined that the ban was lifted. The following description of the effects of moxibustion is based on the these early data for the application of scarring moxibustion[29]; the data indicate that there is a definite need to re-evaluate moxibustion using modern techniques.

White blood cell count

The white blood cell count (WBC) is increased when moxibustion   is performed, with the polynuclear cells (neutrophils, eosinophils, and basophils) in particular being strongly affected. Probably the most famous data are those gathered by *Shimetaro Hara* who applied seven rice grain-sized cones to 10 points in both rabbits and humans. The results, reported in the Fukuoka University Medical Journal in 1929, showed that the rise in WBC peaked at 8 hours after moxibustion and remained high for 3 days; thereafter the WBC diminished to normal levels.

Dr. *Hara* was famous for being a proponent of the use of scarring moxibustion, and applied and burnt cones on *Ashi San Ri* (足三里; ST36) daily on himself. He must have done something right because he went on to become the oldest practising physician in the world, at over

---

[29] Most of the literature cited is written in Japanese. Where possible I have given the English translation of the journal, together with the year of publication.

100 years of age.

Shoichi Tamura published similar results in 1934 (Kanazawa University Medical Journal) and also investigated the amount of moxa necessary to produce the effect. In his study he used four weights of moxa: 0.00017, 0.0005, 0.00075, and 0.001 g/kg body weight; the moxa was applied in one application to several sites on the back. He found that there was virtually no change in WBC for the 0.00017 g group. However, for the 0.0005 g and the 0.00075 g groups, an increase in WBC was noted, reaching a peak over a period of one to 3 days and returning to normal levels over a period of 2 to 12 days. For the 0.001g group, a rapid increase occurring over 3-5 hours was noted.

Macrophages

Moxibustion causes an increase in phagocytosis. According to *Shunji Ota* who published his findings in the Journal of the Japanese Society of Microbiology in 1920, phagocytic activity in rabbits increased 2 hours after moxibustion was applied. The levels stayed high for a period of 4—7 days, reaching a level >2.5-fold those in a control group not receiving moxibustion. More recently, *Eichi Furuya* et al (Japanese Journal of Acupuncture, 1981), using the carbon clearance method, carried out moxibustion on the stomach of mice on 2 points equivalent to the left and right *Ki Mon* (期問; LV14). They used 15 mg of moxa in one application on the 2 points, and showed that the reticuloendothelial system was stimulated, thereby increasing phagocytic activity.

Red blood cell count

The red blood cell count (RBC) is increased by moxibustion. Reports regarding whether the RBC increases are conflicting; however, the majority, headed by the experimentation conducted by the previously mentioned Dr. *Hara*, suggest that in general it does. The variation in the results is probably due to the time frame of the study and the different methodologies used. Dr. *Hara* appears to have favoured long-term daily moxibustion in most of his work; this type of stimulation seems to give more definite results. It would seem appropriate to mention here that the increase in the WBC is an easily noted phenomenon, apparent both to me and fellow practitioners; however, the RBC changes appear to be less definite and appear to require slightly different point selection and moxibustion dosage. Further research is required in this area. Studies could perhaps investigate the effect of moxibustion on the Spleen and Pericardium meridians, which are traditionally connected with blood production, on RBC.

Hematocrit levels

Hematocrit levels are increased by 6 weeks of daily moxibustion. These data again come from Dr. *Hara* and were obtained from a study in which 7 moxa cones were burnt on 11 sites on humans daily for a period of 6 weeks. Surprisingly, during this period no change in the hematocrit was noted; however, one week after moxibustion was discontinued hematocrit levels began to rise.

Platelets

One hour after moxibustion, platelet levels decrease and thereafter increase. These data are based on studies in rabbits (*Takeichi Nagatoya* Medical Association, 1933) in which 6 cones were burnt on each of 4 points on the back; this constituted a single application. After the initial decrease, the platelet count increased one hour later, with levels returning to normal in most subjects within a period of one to 2 days.

Blood sugar levels

Blood sugar levels rise and reach a peak 130 minutes after moxibustion. Based on studies in rabbits, *Tokieda Kaoru* (Japanese Journal of Microbiology, 1926) demonstrated that blood sugar levels 2.5-fold normal levels could be obtained. The levels returned to normal within one to 2 days.

Blood clotting time

Blood clotting time is shortened. In the same study as cited above,

Tokieda shortened clotting time, the effect being most noticeable 30 minutes after moxibustion. Clotting times returned to normal 24 hours later. The data regarding blood sugar levels and blood clotting times remind me of conversations with Japanese war veterans, including practitioners of Oriental and Western medicine, regarding the horrors of war. Food shortages and long marches were often described, and they claimed that the only thing that kept them going was moxibustion. It is possible that the rise in blood sugar levels gave them the spurt of energy required to continue. These war veterans also related how bleeding wounds were stopped using moxibustion or by inserting moxa directly into the wound.

Acid alkali balance

Moxibustion encourages alkalosis and discourages acidosis. A study by *Nagatoya Takeichi* (Journal of the Osaka Medical Association, 1935) in which four points on the backs of rabbits were selected and 8 cones of moxa applied to each, has shown that serum iodate levels decrease immediately after moxibustion, but dramatically increase after 6 hours. Levels returned to normal after 24 hours.

Complement activation

An increase in complement, promoting hemolysis, is observed with moxibustion. *Masatoku Aochi* (Nishin Medical Journal, 1927) conducted studies showing that serum complement levels in rabbits are increarsed and the opsonic effect, which promotes phagocytosis by macrophages, is strengthened by moxibustion. This effect is observed 15 minutes after moxibustion and reaches a peak after 2 to 3 hours; this level is maintained for about one week. The maintenance of serum complement levels suggests that for a healthy immune system, moxibustion should be performed once or twice weekly.

Serum cholesterol

Total cholesterol is reduced with moxibustion. Moxibustion appears to affect fat metabolism in humans. This was investigated by *Hirose*

(Journal of the Japanese Acupuncture and Moxibustion Society, 1971), who burned moxa on the upper and lower back of human subjects and reported that total serum cholesterol levels decreased.

Albumin

Albumin levels initially drop; however, one hour later they rise. *Teramoto Yukio* (Autonomic Nervous System Magazine, 1955) burned 0.1 g of moxa distributed over four points on either side of the neck and lower back of rabbits; two cones were burned on each point. In this way, *Teramoto* showed that although the serum albumin levels initially decreased, an hour later they started to increase.

Globulin

Gamma globulin levels increase with moxibustion. In the same study as described above, *Teramoto* showed that this regimen of moxibustion caused globulin levels, particularly gamma globulin levels, to rise.

Magnesium and calcium levels

Magnesium ion concentrations decrease as calcium ion concentrations increase. *Yoshio Manaka* (Journal of the Japanese Oriental Medical Society, 1958), using human subjects, selected between two and four points and applied seven cones to each daily for one month. The results demonstrated that whereas magnesium ion concentrations decrease ,calcium concentrations increase.

Blood vessels

Initially the blood vessels contract but thereafter dilate, thus improving blood flow. In the same study referred to above, *Yoshio Manaka* performed experiments in which moxibustion was applied to the back of humans. He demonstrated that this resulted in reflex contraction of the blood vessels and therefore a reduction in blood flow, as measured in the extremities during moxibustion. However, 10 to 60 seconds after moxibustion had finished, blood flow returned to normal and then proceeded to increase beyond pre-moxibustion levels.

Gastrointestinal function

Peristalsis is improved with moxibustion. While carrying out research into chronic duodenal and stomach ulcers, *Kazuo Komai* (The Study of Meridians and Points, *Shun Yo Do*; 1939) found that by burning 0.05—0.1 g of moxa in the form of 5cones on *Yu Mon* (幽門; KI21), *Tsu Koku* (通谷; KI20), *Fu Yo* (不容; ST19) in the stomach area and on *Hi Yu* (脾兪; BL20) on the back, peristaltic contraction was greatly increased in amplitude.

Liver function

Liver function is enhanced, pigment discharge is improved, and urobilin is decreased by moxibustion. *Hirose* (Journal of the Japanese Acupuncture and Moxibustion Society, 1969), working with human subjects, measured the total urobilin in the urine and then investigated the effect of moxibustion on Liver function. His findings show that, amongst other things, urobilin levels are decreased with moxibustion.

Internal secretions

Adrenal cortex function is activated with moxibustion. Experiments in which 6 weeks of daily moxibustion were applied and the ability of mice to withstand cold were performed. By monitoring the weight of the phosphate present in the Liver, it was shown that adrenal cortex function is activated by moxibustion.

MECHANISMS OPERATING IN MOXIBUSTION

There are many theories as to how moxibustion works, none of which is without merit. Some of these are described below.

Protein particle theory

The protein particle theory hypothesizes that due to the action of moxibustion on local tissues, proteins are broken down producing the poison histotoxin, which stimulates the immune system to increase antibody production.

Internal secretion theory

In the internal secretion theory, it is postulated that application of moxibustion causes the local release of substances connected with inflammation; this has a direct effect on the humoral regulative processes. In addition, signals transmitted by the peripheral nerves to the central nervous system indirectly affect humoral regulative processes.

The autonomic nervous system

This theory states that moxibustion stimulates the somatic nerves. The central nervous system reacts to this by transmitting signals through (and therefore regulating) the autonomic nervous system.

Nonspecific stress theory

It is hypothesized in the nonspecific stress theory that moxibustion acts as a stressor on the organism and activates the pituitary gland and adrenal cortex, producing an increase in cortisone secretion and thus increased defensive capacity.

3.2   CLINICAL USES OF MOXIBUSTION

Whereas Article 3.1 (Introduction to Moxibustion) considered what moxibustion is, the various techniques that can be used, and the effects of moxibustion on physiological processes, this chapter will describe some of its clinical applications. Thus the two Articles complement each other and should be read in conjunction.

INTRODUCTION

In Japan generally, and definitely in my practice, a treatment involving needling while excluding moxibustion is rare and almost unthinkable. The two techniques complement each other like hand and glove.

A general point to remember is that acupuncture works mainly on the *Ki*, while moxibustion works on the blood, although by working on one you are indirectly affecting the other.

Moxibustion is particularly useful in the following conditions:

1.   Deficient conditions;

2.   Cold and hot conditions;

3.   Chronic conditions;

4.   Immune deficiency;

5.   Low blood pressure;

6.   Chilled conditions;

7.   Skin conditions;

8.   Gynaecological conditions;

9.   Constitutional problems; and

10. Conditions where needling is ineffective.

WHICH TYPES OF MOXIBUSTION ARE MOST USEFUL?

I have found six types of moxibustion to be particularly useful clinically.

Stick moxibustion (棒灸; Bo Kyu).

This can be used on almost any area with no contraindications. It is very useful for balancing right and left, and can also be used daily; I give this type of moxa to patients for self-treatment. For particularly nervous patients, this form of moxa is not so good because they cannot be relied upon to give reliable feedback regarding the degree of heat.

Needle head moxa (灸頭鍼; Kyu To Shin)

This is one of the best types of moxa to use when tonifying in chronic deficiency conditions. It is best used on the back *Shu* points for this purpose. For local treatments, *Kyu To Shin* is excellent when used with deep insertion of needles into joints, for example the "eyes of the knees," *Shitsu Gan* (膝眼; MN-LE-16) or *Kyu Kyo* (丘墟; GB40). In the case of local treatments, *Kyu To Shin* helps blood circulation through the normally poorly supplied joints to hasten recovery. It can be used once or twice daily with multiple applications. If overused, it will cool the joints, and can be used to disperse heat from a painful, inflamed joint.

Needle shaft moxa (灸根鍼; Kyu Kon Shin)

Used when the patient is extremely tired with *Yang* deficiency, and is also great for joint pain where deep Chinese needling is used and the heat is taken deep inside. It is similar in effect to *Kyu To Shin* except that it can be used for both shallow and deep needling; *Kyu To Shin* necessitates deeper needling.

Penetrating moxibustion (透熱灸; To Netsu Kyu)

Can be used to disperse very hard nodules on the Bladder meridian or the governor vessel. It can also be used to tonify the organs using the Bladder meridian. In this case, the cones should be thinner and rolled harder to take the heat deep inside the tissue. However, *To Netsu Kyu* is best used on the legs and hands as part of a root treatment. This type of moxibustion works most strongly on the immune system, and a strong immune system tends to indicate freedom from disease. Although many authorities suggest daily moxibustion using this method, I have found that once, twice, or at most three times weekly is sufficient for most patients. This is borne out by the data shown previously, in which most immunological changes last for about one week after a single application. In addition, unless skillfully done with a low number of cones, daily scarring moxibustion can result in a point that is no longer a useful part of the meridian system, similar to a postoperative scar.

*Heat perception moxibustion (*知熱灸*; Chi Netsu Kyu)*

Chi Netsu Kyu is particularly good for relaxing the upper back when performed in a seated position, although its primary purpose is to disperse stagnant heat trapped on the surface of the skin. This type of moxibustion in the seated position, in which the sympathetic nervous system is tense, is also one of the best methods of relaxing the sympathetic nervous system. *Chi Netsu Kyu* is also excellent for use in the abdominal area, particularly in patients with gynaecological problems.

*Kamaya moxibustion (*カマヤ灸*; Kamaya Kyu)*

Kamaya Mini Moxa - this is basically a small tube with an adhesive at one end and some moxa in it. The moxa is pushed to the top edge of the tube by a plunger supplied with the moxa. The adhesive edge is wetted and the tube is stuck on the skin and the moxa is lit. Contrary to popular belief, the further the moxa is pushed up the tube, the hotter it is.

Caution : there are 2 types the Red coloured Strong type and the Green coloured weak type. It is the latter that I recommend.

It is best used on the back to "melt down" areas of muscular tension and is thus dispersive in nature. It is best not used on the stomach because the heat can be rather harsh. In contrast, the arms and legs do not respond well to *Kamaya Kyu*, due to hair, which can block the heat, or bony areas, which often require more heat. Repeated applications on one spot should be avoided except in special circumstances.

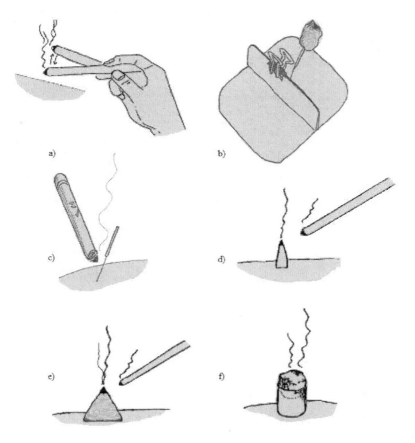

Figure 3-1: Types of Moxa

a) Stick moxibustion (棒灸; *Bo Kyu*); b) Needle head moxa (灸頭鍼; *Kyu To Shin*); c) Needle shaft moxa (灸根鍼; *Kyu Kon Shin*); d) Penetrating moxibustion (透熱灸; *To Netsu Kyu*); e) Heat perception moxibustion (知熱灸; *Chi Netsu Kyu*); f) *Kamaya* moxibustion (カマヤ灸; *Kamaya Kyu*)

Type of Moxa	Back	Extremities	Abdomen	Frequency
Kamaya Kyu	Muscular areas Relatively tense Nervous problems	Rarely used (heat often insufficient)	Best not used	One area of application. daily is OK
Bo Kyu (stick moxa)	Very good. Left/ right imbalance	Very good - left/ right imbalance	Particularly useful on CV8; CV12; ST35	Multiple
Kyu To Shin (needle head)	Best for deep tonification of *Yin*	Sometimes, especially joints and (SP6)	Sometimes	Multiple applications. Best 2-3 times
To Netsu Kyu (direct scarring)	Tendino-Muscular; Governor Vessel	Best on legs, head, and hands as part of root treatment	Sometimes	Multiple cones, treat 2-3 times weekly
Kyu Kon Shin *(needle shaft)*	Good for deep and shallow work	Very good	Excellent	Daily is ok
Chi Netsu Kyu (heat perception moxa)	Particularly upper back in seated position	Sometimes	Excellent	Multiple cones, 2-3 times daily

Table 3-2: Comparison of types of moxa and their use

TONIFICATION AND DISPERSION USING MOXIBUSTION (灸の補寫; *KYU NO HO SHA*)

Scarring moxibustion, contrary to popular belief, can be used to tonify and disperse, similarly to acupuncture. There are various ways to do this. The important points summarized in Table 3-3.

Factor	Tonifying	Dispersing
Wind[30]	Burn cones without fanning	Burn cones with fanning
Number of cones[31]	Fewer	More
Cone Size[32]	Smaller	Larger
Cone Rolling	Softer, loosely rolled	Harder, tightly rolled
Moxa Quality	Better quality	Poorer quality
Ash	Burn cones on top of previous ash	Clear away previous ash before adding next cone
Speed	Slower, leaving a gap between cones	Faster continuous burning

Table 3-3: Tonification and Dispersion

---

[30] This method was first mentioned in the *Ling Shu*, Chapter Fifty One, (靈枢背腧第五十一篇).

[31] This was first mentioned in the *Thousand Emergency Precious Prescriptions* (備急千金要方).

[32] Ibid.

CASES WHERE MOXIBUSTION IS CONTRAINDICATED

According to the Japanese Ministry of Health and Welfare, the following conditions are those in which the practice of moxibustion (and acupuncture) is forbidden:

1. Extremely high blood pressure;

2. Extremely low blood pressure;

3. Cases where there is an extremely high fever;

4. Cases where the disease is unknown or very severe;

5. First 3 and last 3 months of pregnancy;

6. When the patient is intoxicated with alcohol or drugs;

7. When the patient is extremely weak;

8. When the patient is suspected of carrying an infectious disease; and

9. When the patient exhibits mental abnormalities.

If these recommendations were followed, there would be very few patients in which treatment was not forbidden. However, in the initial stages of practice these should serve as guidelines, and when in doubt it is always a good idea to refer patients for a Western medical check-up. In clinical practice as one becomes more experienced, contraindications become increasingly fewer.

FORBIDDEN POINTS FOR MOXIBUSTION

Forbidden areas include the face, the front of the neck, the eyeball, the genital area, pregnant women's abdomens, areas where there is skin disease, areas where there is an acute inflammation, and areas where there are large blood vessels near the surface of the skin. These are again guidelines and are to be kept in mind, particularly when starting to use scarring moxibustion. With experience, "forbidden" comes to mean "to be used with great care," as moxibustion in these areas has a very strong effect.

From a classical viewpoint, the points listed in Table 3-4 are not to be treated using moxibustion. They are listed in order of their frequency of occurrence in 20 classical texts surveyed.

Depending on the classic consulted, forbidden points for moxibustion can number between 24 and 50; therefore the above is a representative list and should not be considered to be definitive. Strangely, the Yellow Emperor's Internal Classic lists only five forbidden moxibustion points: *Gyo Sai* 魚際; LU10), *Ge Kan* (ST7), *Jin Gei* (ST9), *Nyu Chu* (ST17), and *No Ko* (GV17).

It is interesting to speculate why the earliest "bible" (written between 200 BC and the birth of Christ) lists so few, while the later classics list so many. One view is that the experience of succeeding generations swelled the number; another is that after the time of the first classic, standards dropped and more mistakes were made.

Looking at the lists of points, it can be seen that areas such as the face, the nipple, etc are not particularly appropriate for moxibustion (although it can be done). Others are often located in areas where skin creases or folds are present, or where the skin is tight, in which case the scab formed has difficulty healing.

Seki Mon (CV5) is one point that many Japanese acupuncturists omit when using moxibustion in women. I avoid this point in the majority of women. The characters for *Seki Mon* are 石 meaning stone and 門 meaning gate. If this point is treated, traditionally it is said that the woman becomes a "石女" which literally means "stone woman," indicating a barren woman incapable of conception due to hormonal imbalance. *Seki Mon* is the *Mu* point *Bo* (募穴; *Bo Ketsu*) of the Triple Heater meridian, which functionally is connected with the endocrine and

No of Texts	Forbidden Points for Moxibustion
Fifteen	*Fu Fu* (風府; GV16), *Jin Gei* (人迎; ST9):
Fourteen	*Nyu Chu* (乳中; ST17), *Zui I* (頭維; ST8).
Thirteen	*Kyu Bi* (鳩尾; CV15), *Fuku To* (伏兎; ST32)
Twelve	*A Mon* (亜門; GV15), *Yo Kan* (陽関; GB33), *Shi Chiku Ku* (絲竹空; TH23), *Haku Kan Yu* (白環兪; BL30), *Sho Ko* (承光; BL6)
Eleven	*Chi Go E* (地五会; GB42), *En Eki* (淵腋; GB22), *Sei Mei* (晴明; L1), *San Chiku* (攢竹; BL2), *Kei Kyo* (経渠; LU8)
Ten	*So Ryo* (素髎; GV25), *Seki Chu* (脊中; GV6), *Gei Ko* (迎香; L120), *Sho Sho* (少商; Lu11), *Ten Fu* (天府; LU3)
Nine	*No Do* (脳戸; GV17), *Atama No Rin Kyu* (頭の臨泣; GB15), *Sho Kyu* (承泣; ST1), *Ge Kan* (下関; ST7)
Eight	*Shin Yu* (心兪; BL15), *In Shi* (陰市; ST33)
Five	*Seki Mon* (石門; CV5), forbidden for girls, women and pregnant women
One	*Ashi San Ri* (足三里; ST36), forbidden for children.

Table 3-4: Forbidden Points for Moxibustion

lymphatic system. Therefore by stimulating this point, one could reasonably expect changes in hormone levels. The same argument holds for pregnant women, in whom stimulation could cause a miscarriage. In female patients, *Ki Kai* (気海; CV6) or *In Ko* (陰交; CV7) is used instead of *Seki Mon*.

Another point that is worthy of note is *Ashi San Ri* (ST36) , which should not be used in children as it appears to stunt growth. This was attested to by *Misao Takenouchi Sensei* who tried it on his son. The result being that his son's growth rate dropped from normal to the lowest in his class within one year. However, by accident he found that by applying moxibustion to *Yo Ryo Sen* (陽陵泉; GB34) for another problem, his son's growth rate returned to normal.

Another area that is avoided clinically is that around vertebrae T8 and T9 on the Bladder line, which traditionally has no points in it. This is the area where sickness can retreat and leave the body. When a battle is to be fought, unless it is in extreme conditions, there is always an avenue left for the escape of the foe. If this is not done, then instead of an easy victory, the foe will fight to the death because there is no means to avoid conflict. Therefore, although new points and functions have been designated to this area, it is often better to leave it alone.

SOURCES
The texts consulted were as follows:

1. *Ko Te Nai Kei* (黄帝内経) written between 200 BC and the birth of Christ;

2. *Shin Kyu Ko Otsu Kei* (鍼灸甲乙経) written in 282AD;

3. *Sen Kin Ho* (千金方), written in 682AD;

4. *Gaz Dai Hi Yo Ho* (外台秘要方) written in 752 AD;

5. *So Mon Chu* (素問註) written in 762 AD;

6. *Do Jin Yu Ketsu Shin Kyu Zu Kei* (銅人俞穴鍼灸図経) written in 1026AD;

7. *Shi Sei Kei* (資生経) written in 1226AD;

8. *Mei Do Kei* (明堂経) written in l331AD;

9. *Shin Kyu Shu Ei* (鍼灸聚英) written in 1529AD;

10. *I Gaku Nyu Mon* (医学入門), written in 1574;

11. *To I Ho Kan* (東医宝鑑) written in 1611;

12. *Rui Kei* (類経), written in 1624;

13. *Shin Kyu Yo Ho Sinan* (鍼灸要方指南) written in 1686;

14. *Wa Kan San Sai Zukai* (和漢三才図会) written in 1712;

15. *Shin Kyu Cho Ho Ki* (鍼灸重宝記) written in 1718;

16. *Kei Ketsu I Kai* (経穴彙解) written in 1803;

17. *Shin Kyu Setsu Yaku* (鍼灸説約 written in 18ll;

18. *Go Rui Shin Kyu Bassui* (合類鍼灸抜萃);

19. *Shin Kyu I Gaku Tai Ko* (鍼灸医学大綱); and

20. *Sei Ho Shi Mei Do Kyu Kei* (西方予明堂灸経).

For further details, please see *Shin Kyu I Jitsu No Mon (*鍼灸医術の門）by *Sorei Yanagiya* (published by *Ido no Nippon Sha* 1948 in Japanese).

3.3   BURNING QUESTIONS

Q   At school we learned to wipe the area that we had just applied moxa to with alcohol. Is this okay?

The fact that you felt it necessary to ask this question implies that you know that using alcohol to clean the area that moxibustion has been applied to is not acceptable, and you are correct. The application of alcohol is unnecessary and just cools down the area you have been trying to heat up. Don't do it

Q   How should I combine direct moxibustion with my usual treatment routine?

One of the best ways of incorporating moxibustion into your usual treatment routine, especially when starting off, is to choose very carefully 2 or 3 points that are very tender or stiff. Take your time and let the patient lead you rather than feeling that you have to find the points. The upper back and shoulders (normally the second Bladder line) is a good place to start.

Having located the points you want to use, burn one cone on each, partially covering the cones with your finger to cushion the heat. This will have a beneficial effect, and will also get both you and the patient used to direct moxibustion.

Moxibustion should be performed at the end of the treatment and is best done with the patient seated. At the end of the next session, the points can be rechecked and the remaining stiff or painful areas re-treated, this time with two cones each. In this way, direct scarring moxibustion can be introduced gradually and its effect monitored carefully.

A word of warning to those who have sensitive patients: make sure that the cones are rolled as softly as possible and that you burn yourself for at least one week before burning your patients.

Q *How should Kyu To Shin (灸頭鍼; needle head moxibustion)*
be used? How does it work?

Kyu To Shin is useful for any situation where it is advantageous to have
heat deep inside an area. Often it is useful for tonification of *Yin*. This is
achieved by needling deep into a hollow (deficient) area and applying
Kyu To Shin, in which case the heat enters the weak, energy-less areas
through the needle and softens the area. In contrast, it can also be used
for dispersion of *Yin*. For stiff areas, ie, in stagnation of blood or for
nourishing *Ki*, the needle should be inserted down to the stiff area (not
through it) and *Kyo To Shin* applied. This causes the hard area to "melt,"
improving the flow of nourishing *Ki*.

The burning of moxa near the body is also very interesting. The
products of burning moxa are are white smoke and red moxa ember. The
white smoke comparatively *Yin* in nature and rises toward heaven
(*Yang*). The red ember is hot and *Yang* in nature and sinks towards the
earth (*Yin*). This powerful "splitting" of *Yin* and *Yang* occurring near the
body is transmitted through the needle into the body. For any change to
occur in the universe, either internally or externally there must be a
"splitting" of *Yin* and *Yang* from the normal state of equilibrium. When
Kyu To Shin is viewed in this light, it is a powerful signal of change to
the organism. It should also be noted that the practitioner is also
"splitting" *Yin* and *Yang* energies when he moves *Ki* through himself of
through the needle. When this phenomenon occurs, anybody (or anything) nearby will be influenced, even if they are not the object of
treatment.

3.4   *SAWADA RYU*: A TREATMENT STRATEGY

This article outlines some of the unique treatment strategies employed by the famous Japanese acupuncturist *Ken Sawada*, although "moxibustionist" may be a better description because most of *Sawada's* treatment consisted of moxibustion rather than acupuncture. One important thing to remember is that all of his moxibustion was of the direct, scarring type, which I particularly value because it shows that his treatments were geared for efficiency without any frills. When scarring the body, even if the scar is only 2 or 3 mm in diameter, point selection should be more rigorous. *Sawada's* patients objected to being burnt then just as they do now, but due to the efficacy of his treatments they kept coming back. Therefore *Sawada's* treatment strategies, born of a harsh climate, are all the more laudable and therefore worthy of serious consideration.

At the heart of his treatment style is the concept of the all inclusive, overall body regulation method, termed *Tai Kyoku Ryo Ho* by *Sawada*. *Sawada's* martial arts background is reflected in *Tai Kyoku Ryo Ho*, which emphasizes palpation of the body, particularly the lower abdomen or *Dan Tien* (丹田), known as *Tan Den* in Japanese. Interestingly, *Sawada* hardly ever used the pulse for diagnostic purposes, all information being gathered by questioning, touch, and sight.

TAI KYOKU RYO HO – ALL INCLUSIVE TREATMENT METHOD

Basic principles

The aim of treatment is placed firmly on strengthening the *Gen Ki* (元気, source energy) and thus the five *Zang* and six *Fu*. When this aim is achieved, the sickness, whatever its location, will be healed.

Use of theTriple Heater

Gen Ki (source *Ki*) comprises two parts, the prenatal and postnatal, known as the *Sen Ten No Ki* (先天の気; pre-natal *Ki*) and *Ko Ten No Ki* (後天の気; post natal *Ki*). *Ki* is that present at birth and is distributed throughout the five *Zang* and six *Fu*, particularly in the Kidneys. However, in the absence of the postnatal *Ki*, there is only potential without action.

The postnatal *Ki* consists of the *So Ki* (宗気; gathering/ancestral *Ki*), provided by the Heart and the Lungs, the *Ei Ki* (営気; nutritional *Ki*), produced by the Liver and Spleen, and the *Ei Ki* (衛気; defensive *Ki*)(different character same pronunciation), derived from the Small Intestine.[33] The gathering/ancestral *Ki* powers the upper heater (上焦); the nutritional *Ki* the middle burner (中焦); and the defensive *Ki* the lower burner (下焦).

According to the *Sawada* school, the Triple Heater is the means by which *Ko Ten No Ki* (postnatal *Ki*) is absorbed into the organism and combined with the *Sen Ten No Ki* (*prenatal Ki*) to produce activity. *Tai Kyoku Ryo Ho* seeks to ascertain the state of the *Gen Ki* and regulate it accordingly.

Assessing the Gen Ki (元気; source Ki)

As a general rule, *Sawada* would begin by examining the lower abdomen of the patient. This area, known as the *Sei Ka Tan Den* (臍下 丹田 i) or lower *Dan Tien* is the place where "the pulsation between the Kidneys, which represents the life force, the root of the twelve meridians (腎間の動気), is felt."[34] Palpation of this area provides information as to whether the *Gen Ki* is *Kyo* (虚, deficient).[35] Even if the presenting symptoms are mild, if the *Sei Ka Tan Den Gen Ki* is

---

[33] The chyle duct is mentioned in relation to defensive *Ki* by *Sawada*.

[34] See chapter 66 of the *Nan Jing*

[35] A sunken, cold, flaccid lower abdomen lacking in resilience indicates a deficiency in *Gen Ki*. A firm, warm resilient lower abdomen is the ideal.

deficient, recovery will be difficult. However, if the *Sei Ka Tan Den Gen Ki* is in good supply, then recovery will be less difficult even if symptoms are severe. Treatment based on this simple assessment, aims to make the *Sei Ka Tan Den* as full and resilient as possible, and as a result *Gen Ki* will be abundant and recovery from disease will be good.

Meridian and point selection

The *Sawada* school made great use of *Gen Ketsu* (原穴, source points) both for treatment and diagnosis. This is because the Triple Heater *Ki* manifests at and can be regulated at these points. Any pathological change in the five *Zang* and six *Fu* will manifest at these points. The classical inspiration comes from the *Ling Shu* (Spiritual Pivot), although the source points referred to are somewhat different to those used by *Sawada*[36]. The back *Shu* (俞; *Yu)* points are also used extensively, together with the *Mu* (募; *Bo)* points.

A typical treatment pattern

In a typical treatment, the lower abdomen is palpated and found to be lacking in resilience. The cause of the *Gen Ki* (source *Ki*) deficiency is then investigated by palpating the source points and/or the *Mu* points. If, for instance, the Spleen source point *Tai Haku* (太白; SP3) is found to be reactive, the cause of the disease is the Spleen. Therefore, in this case, the *Bo* point of the Stomach, *Chu Kan* (中脘; CV12) is treated; *Ki Kai* (気海; CV6) would also be treated. The patient is turned over and the *Shu* points of the Spleen, Kidneys, and Triple Heater are palpated and treated as necessary. Finally, *Kyoku Chi* (曲池; LI11), *Yo Chi* (陽池; TH4), *Ashi San Ri* (足三里; ST36), and *Tai Kei* (*Sawada* style) (太谿; KI3) on the arms and legs are treated. The treatment is deemed to be

---

[36] The relevant section is chapter 1, entitled *"Nine Needles, Twelve Sources"*. It should be noted that the heart source point is listed as *Dai Ryo* (大陵; PC9) on the Pericardium meridian. The reason for this is detailed in chapter 71, *"Invasive Pathogens"*, where it states that the heart cannot become deficient as this would mean death. Therefore any heart related problem would be treated using the Pericardium meridian. In Japan today, most meridian therapy practitioners do not use the heart meridian at all.

effective when resilience returns to the lower abdomen and the reactivity of SP3 and the *Shu* points disappears.

In addition to treating the relevant meridians, a number of basic points are used for the purpose of overall body regulation. They are:

1. ***Yo Chi*** (陽池; **TH4**). Used often, this is the source point of the Triple Heater meridian and is good for tonifying the lower heater. The left *Yo Chi* in particular is used, and when used in combination with *Chu Kan* (中脘; CV12) it is good for uterine cramps, testicular infection, and tilted uterus. Used often, this is the *Mu* point for the Stomach and represents the middle burner. It is good for any gastrointestinal problems. When used in conjunction with *Yo Chi* (TH4) it is good for tilted uterus.

2. ***Tai Kei*** (太谿; **KI3**). Used often, *Sawada's Tai Kei* is taken to be where the normal *Sho Kai* (昭海; KI6) is located and is used as the source point for the Kidney. It is used for any type of Kidney disease, sore throats, tonsillitis, middle ear infection, asthma, and gynaecological diseases.

3. ***Ashi San Ri*** (足三里; **ST36**). Used often for all types of stomach problems; however, *Ashi San Ri* is not used in patients where there is overproduction of stomach acid. In addition, it is used to regulate nose secretions and to improve vision. From ancient times it has been called "eighth day moxibustion," referring to the widespread folk practice of applying moxibustion to this point for the first 8 days of each month in Japan.

4. ***Kyoku Chi*** (曲池; **LI11**). Often used for preventing suppuration of existing skin problems, *Kyoku Chi* is also used to improve eyesight.

5. ***Te San Ri*** (手三里; **LI10**). Not often used, *Te San Ri* is good for facial paralysis and heavy facial acne. When used for facial

paralysis and heavy facial acne, it should be combined with with *Yo Ro* (養老; S16) to promote faster healing.

6. *Ji Kan* (二間; **LI2**). Used for children's night terror and eye problems including styes.

7. *Ki Kai* (気海; **CV6**). Used often, *Ki Kai* is known as the "sea of *Gen Ki.*" Used also for intestinal problems and chronic appendicitis.

8. *Shin Yu* (心俞; **BL15**). Not used often, when it is *Shin Yu* is used for heart disease and extreme nervousness.

9. *Hai Yu* (肺俞; **BL13**). Not used often, when it is *Hai Yu* is used for patients with poor constitutions, making them liable to catching colds, when it is used in combination with *Fu Mon* (風門; Wind Gate; BL12).

10. *Kan Yu* (肝俞; **BL18**). Used often, especially for nervousness, pale facial colour, insomnia, and eye problems.

11. *Hi Yu* (脾俞; **BL20**). Used in almost every treatment, especially for any digestive problem.

12. *Jin Yu* (腎俞; **BL23**). With *Chu Kan* and *Yo Chi*, *Jin Yu* is probably the most used point in *Sawada's* arsenal. It is used for any type of Kidney problem, but also for skin problems, for instance white patching.

13. *San Sho Yu* (三焦俞; *Shu*; **BL22**). Used for any type of blood/lymph disease and diabetes.

14. *Ji Ryo* (次髎; **BL32**). Used very often, especially for gynaecological problems, male and female sexual organ problems, rheumatism, and stiffness of the back of the neck.

15. ***Shin Chu*** (身柱; **GV12**). Used very often, *Shin Chu* is especially good for vertigo, asthma, the control of epilepsy, and children's diseases such as night terror.

16. ***Yo Ryo Sen*** (陽陵泉; **GB34**). Not used often, but always used for muscular problems, especially of the upper body.

17. ***Ko Sai*** (孔最; **LU6**). Used for reducing pain from haemorrhoids. Taken to be 2 cun down from *Shaku Taku* (尺沢; LU5) at the same level as *Te San Ri* (手三里; LI10).

Getting started

To avoid the trap of getting too far away from clinical practice, I will attempt to make a usable "*Sawada* package" of the above points. Remember this book is not meant to be left on a coffee table in the corner of the room, it is meant to be questioned, sweated over in the clinic, and attested to by the patient.

One criticism of *Sawada's* method made by Japanese practitioners is that it uses too many points for moxibustion. A fair number of points are used, but that was basically all that was done. Moxibustion was not done in combination with a significant amount of acupuncture. Furthermore, this technique originates from a time when drugs were not as freely available and people were not as well nourished as they are today. This meant that a method such as moxibustion to build up the blood and immune system was ideal.

Today, although drugs and nutritional status have improved, the challenges facing our immune systems are in some cases greater than ever before. Thus this is a good time to re-evaluate the incredibly effective role that moxibustion can have. In my experience, when everything else has failed, moxibustion has helped resolve the problem. Inspired? OK, from your next treatment please use the following technique.

Assuming your treatment includes another modality, please incorporate the following set at the end of the treatment session.

1. *Ki Kai* (CV6);

2. *Tai Kei* (KI3 - *Sawada* style - see above);

3. *Chu Kan* (CV12);

4. *Yo Chi* (TH4);

5. *Kyoku Chi* (LI11);

6. *Ashi San Ri* (ST36);

7. *Hi Yu* (BL20); and

8. *Jin Yu* (BL23).

Choose two of these points per session and rotate them each session on a weekly basis. The dosage is seven lightly rolled rice grain sized cones per point.

This type of treatment is of particular benefit for immuno-depressed patients and for those that have reached a plateau health wise. The points have been arranged so that they can be used in numerical order, ie, *Ki Kai* (CV6) and *Tai Kei* (*Sawada* style - see above) may be used in one session, *Chu Kan* (CV12) and *Yo Chi* (TH4) in the next, etc. If one pair is found to be particularly effective, it can be continued; however, use of a single pair of points should not be continued for more than five consecutive sessions before moving on to the next.

3.5 LUNCHTIME MOXIBUSTION CONVERSATION

(Notes from a brief conversation between EO and an *understandent*[37] about moxabusion)

Penetrating moxibustion (透熱灸; To Netsu Kyu)

The important bit is what happens when the heat touches the skin and what happens thereafter. If the moxa cone is hard, it touches the skin and drills right in - very deep and obviously it will disperse the surface – the Defensive *Ki* (衛気; *Ei Ki*). Remenber that in this case we can vary the thickness, the tightness etc of each cone to the condition and task before us.

Heat perception moxibustion (知熱灸; Chi Netsu Kyu).

Actually it is not about touching the skin - it's all going on before then. So actually, if the moxa cone is very hard, the heat moves very slowly towards the Defensive *Ki* and the skin. So actually it is more tonifying of the surface.

"ThinKyu"

(variously *called "SoftKyu or SmallKyu"*) In general this type of *Chi Netsu Kyu* is used on *Yang* Deficient (陽虚) conditions where the intention is to tonify the interior without damaging the surface or resulting in excessive radiation from the surface. The most important issue here is the shape – the diameter – this is the main thing that will tell us whether it will go inside or not. This is primary. Then to a lesser degree, we can consider the density. Yes, if the moxa cone is soft, it will burn quicker and it will affect the Defensive *Ki* less. But if it is falling to bits then it's no good.

---

[37] A term coined by the author to describe a practitoner whose efforts are focused toward **understanding** through learning and practise of the art. The distinction with the term "student" is explored in an Article entitled "Not The Sharpest Knife In The Draw - Speculations On Learning" in Vol III of *A Long Road*.

Stick moxibustion (棒灸; Bo Kyu).

With the stick I can't control the tightness or the density of it but I can control the thickness. The Chinese thick ones, this will all go in the surface – it's a large area of moxa. I don't use that one. *Ikeda Sensei* would say that it is dispersive. However, because of my first teacher, *Takenouchi Sensei*, and because sometimes I find it useful when I don't want the heat to go in too much, but on the other hand I don't really want to do *Chi Netsu Kyu,* then I might use it the thinner Japanese stick moxa. Sometimes I apply this type of moxabustion at the top of the needle – or at the *tip* of the needle – this is called *Kyu Kon Shin*. In this case it goes in a little bit since the needle is there. But it's more efficient, or creates less wastage than the larger one.

Where do we do the Moxa?

Thin-kyu is not applied to the hard areas – it goes in deep – so you obviously don't do this on a hard area – try it – try pushing a thin object deep into a bony hard area of the body (to move to the extreme – then we can apply this thought process to hard indurations in the general flesh too by analogy). On a soft area (deficient) it will sink in to tonify where the deficiency is. By the same logic, larger cones are applied to hard areas – to warm the surface – to allow radiation/ shunting to occur as the Defensive *Ki* is attracted to the area. This should have the effect of softening the hardness.

3.6 MOXIBUSTION MEMOIRS

It all started a long time ago in my first year at Japanese acupuncture school in Tokyo. Those were the days when exams were noisy affairs resembling an Al Capone movie with gunfire in every scene. Indeed, that exam room was my first real taste of the difference between the West and East. The same sombre-faced students, the same official-looking examiners were all there. Everything appeared the same, but once we started, I got a shock. Suddenly, the sound of rapid, staccato gunfire nearly deafened me. After recovering my wits in a carefully controlled and mute way (This was an exam, after all), I realised that the noise was an inherent by-product of writing Chinese characters, or *kanji,* as they are known in Japan. When we write in the West, we slide a pen across the page to create all of our letters and words; in the East, writing *kanji* requires separate strokes, which, when you are in a hurry, means NOISE. On top of that, we were made to use pencils, which made the sound of harried scratching even worse.

Looking back on those days, I think that I had to have been mad, or more politely "gripped by *something*," to have started this unusual enterprise. To start the study of Oriental medicine in Japan was to go to a world away from the 'civil engineering and deep-fried-chips-with-everything' world that I had inhabited and been part of. Anyway, this is quite decidedly another story and I shall not enter this one, at least if I can help it. Back to the story. In the beginning of my studies, I was somewhat handicapped by my lack of language skills, so the practical lessons were the ones I enjoyed and did well in. In what I later realised was part of a time-honoured and natural progression, my massage skills began to develop first, with my favourites being *Anma* (按摩)(lots of unusual fiddly techniques), *Shiatsu* (指圧)(simpler, more direct use of force) and Western massage (lots of oil and powder).

The teachers were of the "old school," which meant in this case, that they wouldn't even consider entering the tatami classroom unless all the shoes (always removed before entering any house in Japan—saves on carpet, I can tell you!) were neatly arranged in rows. As I mentioned earlier, there's far too little ritual in most people's lives, and if there's any at all, it has often been divorced from meaning over time. But here we had ritual with a meaning that was distant enough from this modern world to give a quaint charm to the proceedings, along with a few gentle kicks up the arse to those who lapsed with the shoes.

When I sometimes mention this ritual to my Western (and Japanese) friends in the trade, often they are shocked, bemoan cultural differences, and proceed with vociferous attacks on the Roman Catholic Church, Islam, Buddhism, and the British Royal Family and all it stands for. But they are moaning to the wrong man. I (and others) wanted to learn and was willing to go through the bothersome chore of arranging shoes. This meant, as you may have guessed, that we were also willing to go through the bothersome chore of *learning what our teacher wanted to show us.* Since many people (including many, I hasten to add, who have studied with reputable teachers) seem to be unaware of this fact, let me speak more plainly: it is not *what* you learn, it is the *way* you learn that is of importance. The information you gain is finite; the way you learn will dictate the type and quality of information you obtain both at that time and in the future. Respect for your teacher and your subject are the prerequisites for learning. To those of you reading this who think you know better, what are your results like?

In one lesson, my teacher gave me a bamboo tube that could, he said, be used to regulate the heat of direct- scarring moxibustion. Now at that time, I took great pride (which was unfortunately not matched by my ability) in my moxibustion skills, so I didn't see the use of such a device. I felt I was good enough to do good moxa without it. Although I was very fortunate to have had a number of teachers at my school who were the direct students of *Isaburo Fukaya*, the late, great, famous moxibustionist of Japan, and although they awakened me to the potential of moxibustion from early on, I didn't get into it. It was to moxibustion's younger sister, the slender, silver maiden - acupuncture - that this young man's fancy turned. However, looking back, I think this favouring of acupuncture was also part of a natural progression: after my hands had developed and after I had gained a working familiarity of the body, I wanted to needle it. And by God I did, in all ways and means using everything from long Chinese needles (These were my favourite.) to small intra-dermal needles. No one and nothing was exempt from my obsession. My girlfriends suffered without knowing why, and my classmates suffered, too, although a little more knowledgeably.

Of late, moxibustion has become ever more fascinating to me. There are two reasons. The first and foremost is that I'm encountering more difficult cases than I've ever had before. The second is that, by accident, I discovered what direct-scarring moxibustion feels like when it traverses the thin line between burning and tickling. It's difficult to describe, but let me put it this way: because the feeling is neither burning nor tickling, it actually becomes more than the individual sensations and even more than if they were combined. To put it in Oriental medical jargon, we can say that there's a moxa-stimulation level that isn't enough to arouse the Defensive *Ki* but is just enough to gather *Yang Ki* before it turns defensive.

Unfortunately, moxibustion in general has been receiving a raw deal for too long. Probably most of you who graduated from schools outside of Japan had about three or four hours worth of moxibustion lessons for your whole three-year programme! Moxa education is in such a sorry state that a college I once visited even used one of my articles from some magazine I don't remember as part of their curriculum for a moxa course. Desperation knows no bounds!

But I can't emphasise enough the benefits of studying moxibustion. For one thing, good, solid moxibustion is a perfect antidote to a horrifying trend that has now filtered its way into the acupuncture world, a trend nurtured by the influences of cosmetic-sales techniques and fast food chains. This phenomenon is known as "McDonald's" acupuncture and is as fast and nasty as its namesake.

There are, however, two important differences: McDonald's hamburgers *are* hamburgers and are inexpensive, whereas "McDonald's" acupuncture is misrepresented as Japanese acupuncture and is expensive. In fact, most of the time, the stuff presented in "McDonald's" seminars is more representative of a person than a nation, and if the unfortunate graduates of these seminars ever visit Japan, they'll encounter a rude awakening.

With moxibustion though, you have to take time to roll a cone or two, choose a point carefully, and set fire to the moxa. Now as you, the discerning reader, may have surmised, none of this lends itself particularly well to hard sales techniques or extensive numbers of seminars - or maybe I mean a number of expensive seminars; to hell with it, I mean both. You may be a person who has been to a foreign country to learn moxa for all of three months or so before you decide, in all your wisdom, to teach it, but with moxibustion (and anything else really) your performance will only be of three months maturity. With moxibustion, "howling time" is necessary. This starts by applying moxibustion to your body; suffering the heat late at night, the only time you can find for experimenting; howling at the moon in pain and anguish; and then trying to do better next time. Then after a period of time, you can try it on your colleagues, and then lastly, on your patients. All of this takes time, and unless you are a pyromaniac, it isn't particularly exciting.

CASE STUDY ONE
You are probably wondering why a case study appears here. Simply put, you need to know why I am raving on the way I am!

Condition & History
Female office worker, aged 30 suffering from depression. She had a

history of upper- respiratory disorders. Her older brother passed away unexpectedly at a young age. She was also going through an uncertain period in her life as far as her career was concerned. Added to this was an abortion and relationship difficulties.

She was of medium build and had recently developed a number of pimples around the chin and cheeks. There was pain and resistance to pressure found at *Chu Kan* (中脘; CV12), *Ko Ketsu* (巨闕; CV14), and *Danchu* (膻中; CV17), and there was tightness below the ribs on the right side. Overall, the pulse was wiry with weakness found at the right-medial and left-distal positions. The left-medial pulse was strong, even upon firm pressure, and the right-distal pulse was sunken and in excess.

Considerations

Although the right-distal (Lung) pulse was sunken and in excess, indicating Lung Heat, she had no upper-respiratory symptoms. I surmised that she was basically Spleen Deficiency Liver Excess with a small amount of Heat creeping up from the Liver into the Lungs. The depression slowed the function of the Lungs, impeding the circulation of *Ki*, causing Blood to accumulate in greater quantities in the Liver. This caused more Heat than usual to build up in the Liver, and this in turn caused more Heat to build up in the Lungs.

Treatment

The Spleen was tonified using *Dairyo* (大陵; PC7) and *Tai Haku* (太白; SP3), whilst the Liver Blood was shunted by using *Ko Kan* (行間; LV2). The Lung *Ki* was shunted by simple insertion to *Kosai* (孔最; LU6). This treatment pattern helped her feel a bit more comfortable, but did not make much of a dent on her depression. Her pulse didn't seem to change much either.

After four or five treatments, I remember at one point she was face down, when I looked at her upper back and realised in an instant that her

Upper Heater was totally dysfunctional. I instinctively felt that I had to find a way to move the stuck Heat from her Upper Heater and distribute it to the rest of her body. So I decided to perform direct moxibustion at a level not strong enough to cause even more Heat to stick in the Upper Heater. I chose about fifteen sites on her upper back at points where it was hard and painful on pressure. These points included some found on the Governing Vessel. When I applied direct-scarring moxibustion to all of these sites, I made sure that the cones were smaller than usual (about half-rice-grain size). Further, I cushioned the heat of each cone with my thumb and forefinger to allow the heat to just kiss the skin. With each cone, I checked to see if she felt the heat or not and found that certain sites needed more cones than others. After about ten minutes, I had covered all fifteen sites, and the upper back had loosened up considerably. The patient confirmed this, saying that she felt very comfortable and warm throughout her entire body. I turned her over and checked her pulse. It was totally different. The whole pulse had come to life. The Spleen had come to life. The Liver was unrestrained. And the Lung Heat had gone.

It became clear to me that a number of things had happened. The first thing was that the moxibustion had balanced the left-right, up-down aspects of the upper back. The second thing was that the moxibustion had not caused more Heat to stick in the Lungs, as is sometimes reported classically. What the moxibustion did was cause the function of the Lungs to improve its circulation of *Ki* throughout the body. The patient improved rapidly after that session and is now a normally-adjusted young lady.

"SOFT-*KYU*"

Well, anyone who has spent any time in my clinic knows that I am always experimenting with something, and so it was with the moxibustion I performed on the patient above. I called it soft-*kyu*. After that day, I must have performed it on nearly every patient, whether they were willing or not, suitable or not. I always performed soft-*kyu* on the upper back because I believed that if the Upper Heater functioned properly, it would circulate energy to the rest of the body. The result was that a lot of people benefited. Most of them had had stiff shoulders and necks from cerebral activities, which had caused *Ki* to become stuck in the upper parts of their bodies. Because I monitored the moxa heat and carried out the soft-*kyu* only to the point when a patient felt heat, I didn't have even one case (even in cases with a lot of Lung Heat, i.e., severe asthma) with any worsening of the condition.

The other result was that after about three weeks, my fingers began to ache like a bastard. At night it felt as if metal shavings had embedded themselves in my fingers. I had to find another way of cushioning the heat—it was then that I remembered the tube.

Now, when using no tube and cushioning the heat with your fingers, and when increasing the function of the Upper Heater is the desired effect, you use cones of half-sesame-seed size. In doing so, the heat delicately penetrates the surface of the skin without arousing the Defensive *Ki* too much. The sesame-sized cone gives off an amount of heat that penetrates to the surface layer (*Yang* part) of the Nutritive *Ki*.

Using the tube is a whole different ball game... The tube allows the moxa to effortlessly penetrate deep into the body. It actually cuts off the flow of the Defensive *Ki* to the area where the direct-scarring moxibustion takes place. Remember that the character for Defensive *Ki* is 衛気 (*Ei Ki*) which implies a circling movement around a central precious entity (See Figure 3-1). Also, we know that if Defensive *Yang Ki* does not move, it is no longer functional. Thus the tube is best used when the heat is needed deeper in the body. And it saves your fingers!

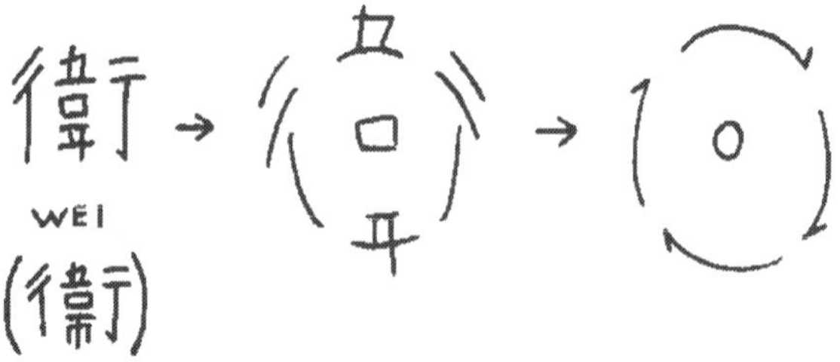

衛行 → (亠口廾) → (0)
WEI
(偉行)

Figure 3-2: Defensive Ki

The meaning of defensive (Japanese: *ei*; Chinese: *wei*), 衛 , as in Defensive *Ki*, '衛気:
The area, '口' is being defended by moving, '行' in a circular manner, '帀' like two
sentries defending something precious.

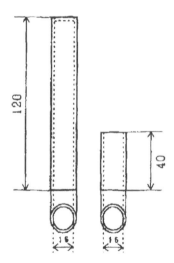

Figure 3-3: Fukaya's Moxa Tubes

Fukaya used two sizes of tube, as shown in this diagram from one of his books[38]. The
larger tube, 120 x 16 mm, was used for applying greater pressure on the point, while
the smaller one, 40 x 16 mm, was used to apply less pressure around the burning
moxa.

---

[38] *Fukaya Isaburo, O Kyu de Byouki wo Naoshita hanashi.* Rev. ed., Sanei, 2000

It was *Isaburo Fukaya* who originally thought up the tube. (See Figure 3-2 and Figure 3-3) Some people think (even in Japan) that *Fukaya* did so to regulate moxa heat. This is, I believe, mistaken for at least two reasons. The first is that it's difficult for me to believe that a man of *Fukaya's* skill and experience (He came up with the tube towards the end of his career.) was unable to make moxa cones that were of the right size and gave off the right amount of heat. The second reason is that if the tube method is tried out in the clinic, the results speak for themselves. Have a look at the next case study and you'll see what I mean.

CASE STUDY TWO

Condition & History

A 34-year-old female fashion designer suffering from dizziness, stiff shoulders, and persistent, nagging lower-abdominal pains. The patient had been examined by a gastroenterologist with no irregularity found. Her gynecologist found three large fibroids. While the location of these was not causing any pressure on the Bladder or Large Intestines, they may have been causing discomfort in the lower abdomen.

The patient was of normal physique with slightly pale skin and nothing significant on the tongue. Overall, the abdomen was somewhat lacking in resilience, except for stiffness and tenderness at *Chu Kan* (CV12) and the right quadrant of the lower abdomen. The pulse was weak, thin, and sunken. The right-medial (Spleen) pulse was a little rough. I suspected a Liver *Yang* Deficiency Syndrome.

Treatment

Touch-needling to the abdomen was performed, followed by tonification of *Tai Kei* (太谿; KI3), *Tai Sho* (太衝; LV3), and *San In Ko* (三陰交; Sp6). This was followed by *Chu Jo Ryu Kyu*[39] (or "triangle-*kyu*", as we

---

[39] *Chu Jo Ryu Kyu* (中条流灸) is an old method of moxibustion that involves measuring the width of a patient's mouth with a piece of string and then using the string to form an

call in it in my clinic) to the lower abdomen with 15 cones on each point. This was done because it was one of my obsessions at the time for dealing with Liver *Yang* Deficiency Syndrome. (It had some interesting repercussions with my patients![40]) For this patient, the dizziness and stiff shoulders seemed to clear reasonably quickly, but the lower abdominal pains seemed to hang on despite my best efforts. I thus decided to try the tube moxa. I palpated the abdomen carefully and found tenderness at *Chu Kan* (CV12), at both left and right *Ten Su* (天枢; ST25), and at a point on the lower right abdomen.

When using the tube, I find it to be more effective if the moxa cones are made twice rice-grain size. So I applied the moxa and found that *Chu Kan* (ST12) needed 5 cones before heat was felt, and upon moxibustion to the other points, heat was felt after about 2. From the way she absorbed the heat from the tube moxa, I instinctively knew it would be effective. So after this, I did very little else during the treatment, just a half hearted root treatment and shallow needles retained at the back-*yu* points (back-*Shu* points in TCM). But this one treatment caused a total cessation of the lower abdominal pain.

---

equilateral triangle. The apex of the triangle is then placed at the middle of the patient's navel, and the two points found at the other two corners are marked on the lower abdomen. These second points then have moxa cones burnt on them, the number of cones corresponding to the age of the patient. So for instance, a 30-year-old woman would have thirty cones burnt on each point; an 18-year-old, eighteen, and so on. This method of moxibustion is famous for treating female infertility.

[40] I found that about 10% to 15% of my female patients fell pregnant. Some were planned. Others had been engaging in certain "family-planning methods" yet fell pregnant after regular triangle-*kyu*. It got to the stage where I had suspicious husbands coming in to see what I was doing to cause such a fertility jump! Not only that, but when it came time for the women to give birth. I was dealing with breach babies, lack of contractions, high blood pressure, and water retention. For a while, my clinic seemed like a mixture between a gynecologist's office and a maternity ward.

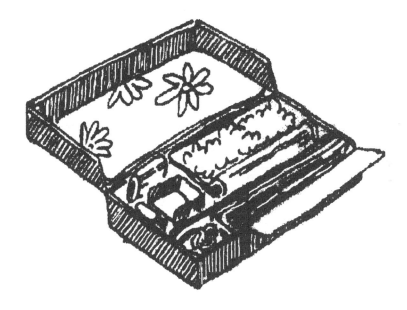

Figure 3-4: Fukaya's Treatment Kit

This is a charming sketch from one of *Fukaya's* books[41] showing the full range of implements he brought to bear in his treatments. They consisted of two bamboo tubes, moxa, incense sticks, a piece of string, a hand-made ashtray/dustbox, a small brush, tweezers, and a pencil. The box itself was made out of cardboard by *Fukaya* himself (quite a dab hand, apparently) and measured 21 x 13 x 3 cm. Armed with this little box and its contents, *Fukaya* treated and cured diseases that fully-equipped hospitals had trouble with.

"TUBE MOXA"

To tell the truth, I was a bit despondent as well as very happy when the tube moxa worked so well. I mean, I had been studying and practising for over a decade with some of the best teachers the art has to offer, and I had a mountain of varied and challenging clinical experience, yet here

---

[41] *Fukaya Isaburo, OKyu de Byouki wo Naoshita hanashi.* Rev. ed., Sanei, 2000

I was getting the best results I had had for a long time by using a simple bamboo tube. It didn't seem difficult enough or bolstered enough by theory.

However, enlightenment appears in various shapes and forms, my friends, and slowly, as I ruminated on this learning experience, insight glowed in me like the rising sun. I began to understand.

Chi Netsu Kyu (heat-perception moxibustion) being thought of as taking heat out and direct-scarring moxibustion being thought of as putting heat in is a load of bullshit! Listen up because I am absolutely (dodgy word) sure of this both theoretically and practically. All moxa puts heat into the system, but depending on the shape of the moxa cones, the heat will go into a different level of the system, giving differing results. Now everything came together: I could see the continuum of moxibustion (All natural phenomena exist in a continuum.) right from the massive *Chi Netsu Kyu* cones to the slenderest of cones for direct-scarring moxibustion.

Also, I thought I remembered reading in *Fukaya's* writings a slight mention about his sometimes varying not just the size but also the thickness of his cones according to where he wanted to put the heat. All of this tied in to make it clear as to what is going on.

I also remembered an article I had read. The writer was confused because one Japanese teacher said that *Chi Netsu Kyu* was tonifying, whilst another stated that it was dispersive. Well, to listen to what some teacher says without thinking about it yourself is a great shame. Doing this immediately puts beyond your reach any possibility of understanding or of further discoveries of your own. But this type of learning is, I'm afraid, rife when it comes to the "mysteries of the East". You are shirking your responsibility for learning if everything comes down to what your teacher says. Probably the only real mystery in learning from the East is that intellectual learning is not the goal, but the beginning, the lowest level of the learning process. The student has to absorb the art psycho-physically and actually demonstrate understanding through practice and not through discussion over tea and cucumber sandwiches.

Anyway, back to the point. When the surface area of the moxa is large, the heat will have little penetrative ability, so will go to the surface, activating the Defensive *Ki* and therefore tonifying the *Yang Ki*. Since one of the main functions of *Yang Ki* is to radiate heat out of the body, putting heat into this level will cause the body to warm up and disperse heat outwards, often with localized sweating, which causes cooling and thus dispersion. This can be likened to being pushed slowly with the open palm. On the other hand, if the cone has a smaller surface area, it activates the Defensive *Ki* less, and with less "friction," the heat penetrates deeper into the body and tonifies the Nutritive *Yin Ki*. Now, *Yin* is contractive, and because the Defensive *Yang Ki* is not so strongly activated with the narrower cones, the heat stays inside, and the body is warmed and therefore tonified. This is like being prodded by a stick.As you might have guessed, speed also has something to do with it: a huge, slow cone probably gives more time for the Defensive *Ki* to react, whilst heat from a smaller cone that burns more quickly is more likely to penetrate. Density of cone is also another factor in the equation, which I will leave you to ponder by yourselves. See Figure 3-4.

Anyway, the use of the tube allows heat from a narrower, smaller cone to penetrate even further because the tube blocks off the Defensive *Ki*, thus eliminating, to a large extent, resistance to the entry of heat into the *Yin* part of the body.

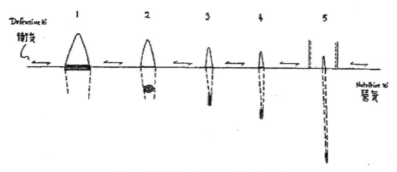

Figure 3-5: Continuum of Moxibustion

1.   Normal-size *Chi Netsu Kyu* affects mainly the Defensive *Ki*.
2.   Smaller-size *chinetsu-kyu* begins to affect the Nutritive *Yin Ki* more.
3/4.   As the diameter of the cones gets smaller and smaller , and as we move
          into direct scarring, scarring, and piercing moxibustion, the heat affects,
          and is therefore affected by, the Defensive *Ki* less and less and moves
          deeper into the body.
5.   When you add the tube, the Defensive *Ki* is locked off completely. This
          means that the heat of the cone does not affect, and is therefore not
          restricted by, the defensive Ki. The heat can therefore move much more
          deeply into the *Yin* areas of the body

CASE STUDY THREE

Condition & History

A 60-year-old housewife with no appetite, dizziness, headaches, lower-back pain, insomnia, and general malaise. I had treated the patient a number of years before for Ménière's disease, and I was shocked at how much weight she had lost. Her skin was pale, almost gray, and she was very thin and almost grim-looking.

The patient had a history of autonomic nervous system disorders, which in everyday terms, means that she was very prone to stress. Since I had last seen her, she had developed this state to a fine art: she was on twelve different medications, including of course, a medicine for the gastric side effects from the other medications. Plus, she had three different prescriptions from her herbalist, one of which, interestingly enough, he convinced her to buy because it cured his cat's hemorrhoids. Her white blood cell count was way below average.

Her lower abdomen was weak, and there was resistance and pain upon pressure at *Ko Yu* (肓俞; KI16), *Sui Bun* (水分; CV9), *Chu Kan* (CV12), and *Ko Ketsu* (CV14). There was some Heat in the chest.

Her pulse was weak, sunken, and rough, with the greatest deficiency felt upon firm pressure at the right-medial and left-distal pulses. The left-medial pulse was also weak, but this pulse seemed to have something within it that did not disappear with pressure.

There was no real coating, and the tongue was rather large for her body.

Considerations

The symptoms and pulse indicated that she was Blood deficient, and the abdomen showed that there was Heat in the chest, probably due to the amount of medication she was on. Both sides of her upper back between the shoulder blades were like strips of wire stretched taut, parallel to the spine. Although this tightness and the pulse indicated Liver Excess, her overall condition was so weak that any dispersion had to come a lot later. The first thing was to work on the Spleen Deficiency to get her appetite back and get some blood into her system.

Treatment

It is always interesting when you begin to work with a patient who you treated many years before because you can see if you have improved or not, or at least if the patient notices any difference. I began by slowly applying touch-needling to *Chu Kan* (CV12), *Ten Su* (ST25), and *Kan Gen* (CV4), then waited for her *Ki* to respond. At this time, my needle was no longer a needle, but a warm, soft thing like a furtive magnet, patiently waiting in the churning waters of her existence for the metallic fish of her life force to bite—or something like that. Her pulse improved immediately, becoming fuller and more lively.

I then tonified *Nai Kan* (内関; PC6) and *Ko Son* (公孫; SP4), and followed with tube moxa to the abdomen at *Ko Yu* (KI16), *Sui Bun* (CV9), *Chu Kan* (CV12), and *Ko Ketsu* (CV14).

Then I had a look at her back and chose a number of sites on the upper back, *Hi Yu* (脾兪; BL20) and *Jin Yu* (腎兪; BL23), for tube moxibustion. Her upper back could not adequately be described by the word "concrete". But her underlying weakness absolutely prohibited any dispersal.

Thus I began the tube moxibustion, and after about two or three cones, I noticed an interesting phenomenon. Under the area of the cone, there was a red mark like the after-effects of cupping, only on a miniature scale. I noticed that this occurred on every point except the Kidney back-*yu* points. Looking at the redness, I realised that the stimulation would cause a rather heavy load on her system, so I stopped the treatment after the tube moxibustion. I told her that she would feel rather sleepy that day and that she should have an early night. I also asked her to come in once a week for a full course and two other times each week for just the tube moxa. I was lucky because she felt very pleasant after the moxa and agreed to the plan. Within three weeks, she regained her appetite, began to put on weight, and was sleeping better. Her headaches still appeared occasionally, but in general, she had more resilience.

"CHAMPAGNE-*KYU*"

Yes my friends, here was another insight handed to me by one of my patients. The redness was caused by the moxa dilating the blood vessels, and the cupping effect was induced by the tube. I exaggerated the effect by holding the tube over the burning cone for longer periods than usual to create more of a vacuum effect before pulling the tube away some- what smartly, in order to get a popping sound.

The sound actually became quite popular, and became even more so when I gave it the name champagne-*kyu,* as it resembled the sound of a champagne cork being popped. Whenever possible, we performed champagne-*kyu* with cork-popping aplomb.

Anyway, with this type of moxa, I could see that by quickly placing the tube over the cone, waiting until the cone is almost burnt down to the bottom, and quickly pulling the tube away, thus exaggerating the vacuum effect, the technique becomes dispersive. This procedure can be contrasted to a slow placement of the tube over a three-quarter-burnt cone, with a slow, relatively early removal of the tube so as not to cause a vacuum.

The great thing about this champagne-*kyu* type of dispersion is that heat energy is first given to the blocked area before the mini-cupping effect is brought into play. So with champagne-*kyu,* because of the concentrated heat and the small size of the tube, there is no real risk of chilling the body, as with normal cupping.

Of course, as you may have guessed, over the next month I used champagne-*kyu* on anybody who came into my clinic. In one instance, someone who was merely waiting for another patient to come out of the treatment area became a target, such was the single-mindedness with which I applied myself to the task. I noticed that paler-skinned people with chronically stiff tissues (but not necessarily Blood Stagnation to the extent that it showed in the abdomen) seemed to be the type who responded with the mini-cupping mark when "champagned".

Another thing that we can assume is that champagne-*kyu* is okay, if not good, for conditions where there is Lung Heat.

At the same time, I just happened to be reading one of *Isaburo Fukaya's* books, and there, in one small section, he made mention of the phenomena! He had been treating a chronic asthma sufferer who had had the problem for twenty years or so, and on the upper back, he noticed the mini-cupping phenomena. He said that the tube moxibustion helped to remove Stagnant Blood.

This was good to know for a number of reasons, the first being that I had unwittingly followed in the steps of the great *Fukaya* and come up with the same type of conclusion. Yeah, I know what you're thinking: if I had read his stuff more thoroughly beforehand, I could have saved myself a lot of time and trouble. But then my friends, I would have had the *information* but not the *research tools*, the method to make my own discoveries. I am not interested in information *per se*, but rather the method, or the *way*.

SUMMARY

Learning this art is more about knowing the philosophy and methods from a clinically experienced teacher and less about gaining information from seminars and books.

Emphasising the former will allow you unlimited progress at your own pace and style. Emphasising the latter will not only *not* allow this development to occur, but will encourage dependence on yet another boring book or seminar from third-rate practitioners.

3.7 *O KYU* (お灸) – A CASE HISTORY

The patient was a young boy of 14 who decided to cut the toe nail of his big toe because it was making holes in his socks. An admirable intention but the result of this was that the nail on the inside (Liver meridian side) was cut too short and began to dig into the flesh. Added to this was a demanding sports schedule combined with the heat of summer. After ten days he developed a grotesquely large and inflamed big toe which prevented him from doing sports and even wearing normal shoes.

Examining his toe, there was a lot of pus oozing from the constantly inflamed nail bed inside. To get a real recovery, we would be talking about the nail growing out again and not pressing on the flesh but something had to be done before that about the inflammation.

Direct scarring moxibustion is not a favourite amongst young boys, young girls, older boys or older girls for that matter but this was a case where I felt that it would be most effective. I chose three points ringing the infected area and did 5 cones of half rice grain size moxa on each point. The next day there was a slight improvement. The same treatment was carried out on the second day with a marked reduction in pain.

The inflammation was improved but the problem itself showed no signs of resolving itself. I decided to see how things would develop over the next few days. Three days later the toe was less painful but looked basically the same. I decided to work on the basic problem now rather than the inflammation. The basic problem was located on the Liver meridian. I palpated the fire point of the Liver meridian *Ko Kan* (行間; LV2) and found it to be very painful upon pressure. This would be the entry point into the Liver meridian and the toe. The nature of the point I was using would be such that it would tonify the fluids of the Liver and therefore clear up the cause of the inflammation. Or something like that. In any event, I decided that I wanted to put a lot of *Ki* into the *Yin* and tonify the *Ei Ki* (榮気; nutritional *Ki*). So I chose to do a large number of thin, thread like cones to allow the heat to go into the *Yin* "without injuring the *Yang*".

So it was that I performed about 50 thread like cones on *Ko Kan* (LV2) on the affected side only. The size of the cones meant that I was able to get away with that large number that I felt was necessary to do the job. It appeared to be an effective strategy because after about the 30th cone the big toe and only the big toe began to glisten with sweat. It appeared that the waste that had been stagnant in the toe was now being washed out by the sweat pouring out locally. This was in line with my objective of tonifying the nutritional *Ki* which moved the blood more efficiently causing the waste to be excreted. Rather than just stick to a prescribed number of cones, I also monitored the pulse and when it appeared to be full and flexible all over, I decided to call it a day. This was at about the 50th cone mark.

The next day the toe had changed nicely. The day after that it was almost normal size and was a lot softer all over. I asked the boy to do some squats to keep the blood moving through the legs. Two days later, the toe looked almost normal.

When moxa is used, you should be clear about what you want to do. In this way *Chi Netsu Kyu, To Netsu Kyu, Kamaya Kyu, BoKyu* can all be effectively utilised[42].

To Netsu Kyu (透熱灸) or penetrating moxibustion is aimed at the Blood or Nutritional *Ki* (榮気; *Ei Ki*). This means that the cones should be as thin as possible to target this and only this. In this way the Defensive *Ki* (衛気; *Ei Ki*) is not harmed and the effect is greater. So naturally it should be as thin as possible. This also means that there is a very small scar which in this day and age is important.

---

[42] See Articles 3.1 and 3.2 for details of these techniques.

3.8 TWO SIDES OF A MOXIBUSTION COIN

Things often occur in pairs (left and right, day and night, man and woman...). Now consider the following pair of areas in the body: the lowest part of the trunk in the front and the highest part of the trunk at the back. This pair of areas is where we'll focus our discussion of two moxibustion techniques: *Chu Jo Ryu Kyu* (中条流灸) and *Hachi Yo Ketsu Kyu* (八曜穴灸).

CHU JO RYU KYU (中条流灸)

In the article titled "Moxibustion Memoirs" included in this Chapter, I mentioned that *Chu Jo Ryu Kyu* (a technique that I dub "triangle moxibustion", or "triangle-*kyu*"), applied to the lower abdomen can be used for lower-back pain, female sterility and for any problem related to Liver *Yang* Deficiency Syndrome. The technique is effective because it puts *Yang* energy (moxibustion heat) into the lower *Dan Tien* (丹田), or "*Tan Den*", as it is known in Japanese. There are a number of *Dan Tiens* in the body, but the reason the lower *Dan Tien* gets so much attention is that it is located in the most *Yin* part of the trunk, i.e., the lower, front part. In this *Dan Tien*, if *Yang* energy can be collected, a lot of energy can be created for the whole body. This is because *Yang* energy has a tendency to rise outwards and upwards, and if it is kept inside and downwards, these opposing forces give rise to life energy.

At this juncture, I guess it's a good idea to look into what the word "*Dan Tien*" actually means. The character for *Dan*, 丹, is often translated as "medicine," and the character for *Tien*, 田, means "field." The question that springs to mind is why the character normally used for medicine, 薬, wasn't used in this compound. The reason is that *Dan* is referring to a special type of medicine, in fact, the raw material for all other medicines. The other thing is that *Dan* is connected with the colour, "red," and represents the substance formed by the mixing of mercury and sulphur: cinnabar, a red mineral. The character for *Dan*, is actually derived from the image of a well, 井, dug in the earth with something exposed in the well during the digging process. That exposed something is cinnabar. So the character for well, 井, with the concept of cinnabar incorporated, gradually became the character for *Dan*, 丹.

It's important to note the significance of the idea of "well" in the character for *Dan*. In ancient societies, and in those of today that live close to nature, wells were intimately connected with life. Indeed, no well meant no chance of survival. The idea of "cinnabar" is also important. Outside the human body, we can think of the combination of the silver-coloured, liquid mercury and the brittle, yellow sulphur leading to cinnabar. For inside the body, this combination can be thought of as a metaphor for combining *Yin* and *Yang* in the depths of the body cavity (well) in the lower abdomen to produce true *Yang*.

The character for *tien*, 田, (or *den*, in Japanese), means "field," normally a cultivated one. In Japan, the meaning is limited to "paddy field," the place where rice (the staple of the diet in the East), or nourishment, is cultivated. Thus, the *Dan Tien* can be thought of as the location where the raw material for nourishment of the individual can be found.

Treatment of the Tan Den (丹田; Dan Tien)

Anyway, having said all the above, we now need to know how we can favourably influence this area to help the patient with disease. Well, probably the best thing is for an individual to influence his or her own *Dan Tien* by utilising the mind and breath, but this is difficult and takes time even for those who are healthy. Fortunately, practitioners can help by means of *Chu Jo Ryu Kyu*, or triangle-*kyu*. This involves measuring the width of a patient's mouth with a piece of string and then using this length of string to form an equilateral triangle. Then, moxa is burnt on the two points below the navel corresponding to the two corners of the equilateral triangle when the triangle is placed with its apex at the centre of the navel (See Figure 3-6).

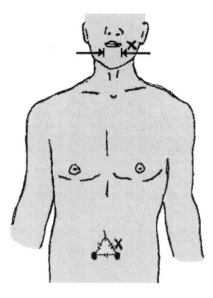

Figure 3-6: Location of Chu Jo Ryu Kyu

Traditionally, the number of cones burnt is equal to the patient's age, so an eighteen-year-old would have eighteen cones burnt, whilst a forty-year-old would have forty cones. Burning cones traditionally refers to burning the moxa directly onto the skin, which unfortunately, can be a little bit harsh. I've adapted (I hate to do this normally.) this technique to today's conditions by using small, thin *Chi Netsu Kyu*, the number of which is determined by the change in the pulse. The moxa should be performed until the pulse changes from a sunken, weak one into a fuller, stronger pulse. At this point, the moxibustion should be stopped because if continued, the pulse will actually start to weaken. The reason for this is that *Yang* Deficiency means that there's not only a lack of *Yang Ki* (in this case, Blood), but also an inability to hold the *Yang* and stop it from leaking out.

When doing *Chi Netsu Kyu* in the case of *Chu Jo Ryu Kyu*, it's extremely important to roll the moxa as softly as possible -just enough to maintain the cone structure - since small, hard, dense cones will disperse instead of tonify. This is because hard cones result in a sudden, searing heat, which activates the Defensive *Ki*, which in turn will not allow the heat to penetrate. Softer cones give a slower, kinder heat that the body does not resist, thus not activating the Defensive *Ki* so much, resulting in a deeper, more penetrating heat sensation. Also, for very *Yang* deficient patients, I ask them to indicate to me the moment just before the moxa feels hot. This is to avoid any chance of dispersion.

If this technique is done correctly, the patient will experience, as well as a favourable change in the pulse, a deep sensation of warmth that stays with him or her during and after the treatment. Women often describe the feeling as being like their uterus was warmed up from the inside. When I had the procedure done, it felt as if my prostate were warmed from the inside. I was curious because I had never felt this before with the more usual methods of warming the lower part of the abdomen with moxibustion, such as salt moxibustion to the navel and needle-head moxibustion to *Kan Gen* (関元; CV4), to name but a couple. I also never got the same clinical results as I did with the triangle-*kyu*. After some thought, I realised this was because of the nature of this *Dan Tien* : It's a spreading field of *Yang Ki*, which has as its nature the tendency to spread outwards and up. This means that any attempt to force heat in on this already outwardly going Heat from the *Dan Tien* will give less than optimum results.

Now is perhaps a good time to talk about *chakras*. Some people think that they're something different from concepts in Oriental medicine—the "Indian" approach. But for me, I believe that as both Ayurvedic and Oriental medical traditions are looking at the same body, they're bound to encounter the same phenomena, though the areas on which they focus as well as their method of expression may be slightly different. Anyway, we can consider *chakras* to be pools of *Yang* energy that tend to accumulate in deep or shallow cavities and on or under projections. Because *Yang* energy has a tendency to spread out and up when it pools, rather than forming a discrete point, it'll form a spherical shape. This is, I believe, the *chakra* phenomenon.

HACHI YO KETSU KYU (八曜穴灸)

While *Chu Jo Ryu Kyu* is done on the lowest part of the front of the trunk, *Hachi Yo Ketsu Kyu*, the second side of our moxibustion coin, is done on the upper part of the back, around the point *Dai Tsui* (大埴; GV14), to be precise. As we know, *Dai Tsui* is the gathering point for the *Yang Ki* of the body. However, in direct contrast to the *Dan Tien* below the navel, *Dai Tsui* is located not in a *Yin* cavity on the lower part of the front (*Yin*), but on a *Yang* projection on the upper part of the back (*Yang*). The area around *Dai Tsui* therefore behaves very differently from this *Dan Tien*. If the lower *Dan Tien* is useful for storing *Yang Ki*, then the area around *Dai Tsui* is useful for radiating *Yang Ki* out of the body. In fact, radiating *Ki* out from this area is probably essential; otherwise, a lot of this action would have to be done from the head, which is okay, but when above a certain level, this action would result in headaches, high blood pressure, tinnitus and other ailments. While thinking about this area one day, I just happened to glance at one of *Isaburo Fukaya*'s books[43], and there it was: Moxibustion to eight points surrounding *Dai Tsui*. It was love at first sight!

In *Fukaya*'s introduction to his book, he stated that moxibustion to these eight points, the *Hachi Yo* points, is amazingly effective for symptoms connected with melancholy, feelings of hatred, Heat, Cold and *Ki* disturbances. It's also effective for chronic vomiting, including that connected with stomach cancer.

Location of the Hachi Yo points

The eight points are located by measuring, from *Dai Tsui*, one *cun* in each of eight directions: namely vertical, horizontal, and diagonal (at the

---

[43] *Fukaya Isaburo, Okyu de Byoki wo Naoshita Hanashi* (Discussions of Curing Disease with Moxibustion). *Shinkyu no Sekaisha*, 1967.

midpoints of the horizontal and vertical directions). This gives the shape as shown in Figure 3-6.

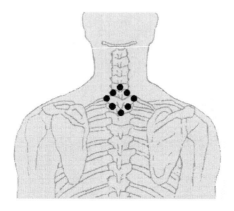

Figure 3-7: Location of the Hachi Yo points

Some of you will recognise this diamond pattern as similar to the shape created by connecting *Shin Chu* (身柱; GV12), *To Do* (陶道; GV13) and *Fumon* (風門; BL12). It's my belief that this shape, lower than the *Hachi Yo* points, was a recognition by past masters that when *Yang Ki* gathers at a location (*Dan Tien*), it cannot be defined or restrained at a given area or spot. However, I believe that the location of this *Dan Tien* is subject to the structure of an individual. In the past, when probably over 90% of the Chinese population were rural workers, it seems possible that their backs became stooped over from labour, thus meaning that the part of the back that stuck out the most (and where the *Yang Ki* gathered) was probably lower down the back than *Dai Tsui*.

Just out of interest, the point, *E Yo* (会陽; BL35), meaning "meeting of *Yang*" and commonly thought of as being part of the Bladder meridian, is referred to in the "Elucidation of the Fourteen Meridians" (十四経発揮) as being part of the Governor vessel. This may seem surprising, but when we think about it, if there's a point, *E Yin* (会陰; CV1), meaning "meeting of *Yin*" on the Conception vessel, then it's conceivable that a corresponding "meeting of *Yang*" exists on the Governor vessel. One of my first teachers, *Misao Takenouchi*, first brought this to my attention, but many people seem to have ignored this idea. Further, rather like the area around *Dai Tsui,* there's a collection of *Yang* energy that bulges out at *E Yo*. At the time of writing, I'm experimenting with this area.

Type of Moxibustion[44]

Direct-scarring moxibustion is recommended in *Isaburo Fukaya*'s book[45] (where he discussed moxibustion to the *Hachi Yo* points), but as with *Chu Jo Ryu Kyu*, I've replaced this technique with small, thin *Chi Netsu Kyu*. The difference between the two is that for *Hachi Yo Ketsu Kyu*, the *moxa* can be rolled a little tighter because we want to promote the radiation of heat out of this area. We don't want to put it in. Also, I instruct the patient to wait until the moment the moxa actually is hot (as opposed to the moment just before the moxa feels hot) before signaling me and telling me so.

Case 1

Symptoms & History: 55-year-old housewife suffering from low-grade fever and weakness for the three weeks prior to treatment. There was frequent urination and a feeling of cold despite the low-grade fever (as measured by thermometer).

The patient had been feeling unwell with a cold and fever for a week before visiting her doctor. The doctor prescribed antibiotics, which the patient took for seven days. This treatment seemed to bring the fever down, but she lost her appetite and began to develop a cough, so she returned to the doctor and was given a different antibiotic. With this second treatment, the cough improved, but the low-grade fever returned along with poor appetite and general weakness.

---

[44] See Article 3.1 entitled "Introduction to Moxibustion and Article 3.2 entitled "Clinical Uses of Moxibustion"

[45] *Fukaya Isaburo, Okyu de Byoki wo Naoshita Hanashi* (Discussions of Curing Disease with Moxibustion). *Shinkyu no Sekaisha*, 1967

There was a grayish tinge to the whole body, including the face. The pulse was floating and rather rapid, and when pressed, very deficient, especially in the two proximal positions. The abdomen was generally flaccid, with a hollowness below the navel. There was no real Heat in the chest.

Treatment: The patient was treated with only moxibustion. Firstly, triangle-*kyu* was performed on the lower abdomen. Nine, soft, small cones of *Chi Netsu Kyu* were burned, resulting in a fuller pulse. After this, the patient was turned over and *Hachi Yo Ketsu Kyu* was performed on the upper back/neck.

After the treatment, the patient was sent home with the explanation that she was not strong enough to receive any needling or massage and with the recommendation that she should take it very easy. Two days later, she returned to the clinic looking much better, reporting that the night of the first treatment, she developed a high fever with sweating, after which her temperature returned to normal. She continued to be a bit weak, but her appetite had returned and her facial colour was better. Two treatments later, she was back to normal.

Considerations: The patient was suffering from Kidney *Yang* Deficiency, which meant that the lower Heater had to be warmed up before anything could be accomplished. In fact, it was this weakness that was slowing down the recovery process. Kidney *Yang* Deficiency can often occur after poor treatment of a cold or fever when someone is already constitutionally lacking in *Yang*. After warming the lower Heater, it was necessary to open the function of radiation of Heat from the upper body using *Hachi Yo Ketsu Kyu*. The two phases of treatment thus resulted in recovery. It's sometimes necessary to follow this two-stage process in very weak *Yang* deficient patients.

Case 2

Symptoms & History: A thirty-year-old female with constant fever for the three days prior to treatment. At first the patient had a normal cold with chills and fever. She felt better and returned to work after two days and, as often happens, was extremely busy. This caused the chills to disappear and the fever to remain.

The patient appeared to be full of energy and felt hot to the touch, basically all over. She was thirsty and suffered from constipation.

She was a bit hot and sweaty all over. Her facial complexion was good).

The pulse was full, smooth and a little fast. It was difficult to discern the deficient pulses. Her abdomen was swollen and hard all over.

Treatment: For this patient, there was no need to put any more energy in; rather, help was needed in radiating the energy out. Therefore moxibustion was applied, not to the lower abdomen but to the upper back/neck area in the form of *Hachi Yo Ketsu Kyu*. I decided to apply *To Netsu Kyu* (direct-scarring moxibustion) using half-rice-grain-sized cones. I applied the first round, but because the *Hachi Yo* points are deliberately not located on normal acupuncture sites, the patient felt the moxa to be very hot. I therefore covered the cones to lower the heat and dropped the size down to quarter-rice-grain-sized cones. After the second round, there was a red "ring of fire" around the point, *Dai Tsui* (GV14). Literally within seconds, sweat just poured out of the patient. Well, when I say, "poured," perhaps I should say, "seeped out" from all over the body. I was stunned, as was the patient, but my initial reaction was quickly replaced with chagrin as I realised that I'd have to change all the sheets. Anyway, I toweled the patient down and sent her home. Her parting words as she left were, "*Sensei*, I feel lighter and clearer." That evening, I received a phone call from her reporting that she had had a bowel movement, that her fever had dropped and that she felt very relaxed.

Considerations: This was probably a case of Spleen *Yin* Deficiency with Stomach Excess. I could have gone the normal root of applying a root treatment, but I was in my research mode (Another way of putting it: I was playing with my new choo-choo toy), so I decided to first try just the moxa. At least in this case, the result speaks for itself.

Case 3

Symptoms & History: A 36-year-old female office worker with Alopecia totalis, sciatica of the right leg. All around the same time, the patient had a number of significant events happening in her life. She was a chronic sufferer of lower-back pain, and with the extra stress, the pain had become worse. Further, her hair had fallen out in tufts.

She was generally tired and slept poorly. There were soft stools during menstruation. She was underweight, had a reasonable complexion and had large eyes compared to the rest of her face.

The pulse was generally weak and sunken, with a little roughness in the Spleen position. Generally speaking, this was unremarkable, although there was some tightness at *Chu Kyoku* (中極; CV3). The tightness was thought to be due to chronic Kidney Deficiency that had given rise to Heat lodged in the Bladder, which caused the sciatica.

Treatment: The patient was treated for Liver *Yang* Deficiency Syndrome. Triangle-kyu was performed on the lower abdomen (seven, small, soft *Chi Netsu Kyu* cones) and a root treatment was performed using contact-needling to *Tai Kei* (太谿; KI3) and *Tai Sho* (太衝; LV3). This was followed by light needling to the Gall Bladder meridian and the entire back.

The patient remarked that, after the first treatment, she went home with a distinct feeling of warmth in her lower abdomen. One week later, the second treatment was carried out and consisted of much of the same as the first. By the third treatment, the sciatica had improved, and by the fifth treatment, the size of the bald areas of the scalp had begun to recede. After 15 treatments at a pace of once a week, the sciatica and alopecia had disappeared. The patient now comes in at a pace of once a month to maintain her health.

Considerations: The patient was originally Kidney deficient, but due to extra stress, she became Liver *Yang* deficient with emphasis on the Kidneys. As well as the pulse and other symptoms, her big eyes were also a factor in choosing the syndrome. Eyes that are relatively big indicate a constitution that should have a lot of Blood in the Liver, i.e., a Liver Excess constitution. Thus a Liver *Yang* Syndrome treatment would start to put Blood into the Liver and help nudge the patient bit by bit back to her constitution. Triangle-*kyu* to the lower abdomen served two purposes. The first was to get the lower Heater to start firing again, hence helping the middle Heater as well (Liver *Yang* Deficiency means that both the lower and middle Heaters are chilled). The second was to use the moxibustion as a sort of indirect local treatment to treat the sciatica. In any case, this moxibustion was indispensable in helping this woman get back on her feet.

3.9 ON PENETRATING MOXIBUSTION (透熱灸; *TO NETSU KYU*)

EO: So here I want to go in without damaging the surface – so it's a very thin insertion. And it's a little harder which will take it in.

TS: What are you trying to achieve by going in deep with the heat here?

EO: Well – there is blood stuck in this meridian. It's stuck at the blood level. So I want to tonify the blood and the blood should move.

TS: Could you do this with *Kyu To Shin* (Needle Head Moxa) also?

EO: Well – you could do it to some extent. But the *Kyu To Shin* is actually less malleable than this to some extent. With this I am actually making the gun at the time I am going to shoot it. It's the same concept, but with the penetrating moxa we can fine tune it.

3.10 THE SPIRIT OF MOXIBUSTION: *ISABURO FUKAYA* AND *KEN SAWADA*

INTRODUCTION

My experience of the dramatic effects of moxibustion on fever led me to look again at moxibustion and its place in the overall treatment strategy. Reviewing the literature, two main figures stood out: *Ken Sawada* and *Isaburo Fukaya*. *Ken Sawada* is well known[46], but *Isaburo Fukaya* less so.

Not only were the methods and points that *Sawada* and *Fukaya* used for various diseases of interest, but the spirit of investigation, originality, and determination they brought to their practice was impressive. In an effort to convey the enthusiasm that their work stimulates, a few of their ideas and treatment strategies are given below, together with some comment. The purpose of this is not just to be informative, but hopefully to inspire and encourage your own process of discovery in the clinic, benefiting both your patients and yourself.

I was fortunate enough to be tutored in moxibustion by a disciple of *Isaburo Fukaya*. This gentleman loved to drink and avoided diabetes by applying direct scarring moxibustion especially to *Ashi San Ri* (足三里; ST36). I remember that a part of each lesson involved one of his students (usually me) doing moxibustion on this point for him. I recall the contented, satisfied look that spread over his face as the cones sunk their heat into his body, as well as how healthy he was (I believe he was 70 years old at the time) all year round and how solid was his grasp of moxibustion treatment. However, it was not until I began to practise clinically full time and encountered difficult cases that I really began to appreciate what moxibustion can do.

---

[46] More information about *Ken Sawada* and his treatment strategies can be found in Articles 3.4 and 3.6

One interesting point that both *Sawada* and *Fukaya* identified is that the tender points for moxibustion appear to come in threes in the shape of a triangle. This was first hinted at in a text known as *Mei Ka Kyu Sen* (名家灸選; Famous Moxibustion Selections) by *Wa Ki Tsui Ryo*, written at the end of the Edo period.

Outlined below are *Isaburo Fukaya*'s *"Ten Rules of Moxbustion"* and his treatment strategy for asthma, together with my commentary. The asthma treatment strategy is particularly interesting because it gives no pathology or physiology but is very effective. The selection of points reveals the work of a highly accomplished practitioner and, if interpreted correctly with an understanding of the syndrome involved, can be used to even greater effect. It also illustrates an important aspect of direct scarring moxibustion therapy: treating consecutively for a number of days and then allowing a rest period during which the body can react to the stimulus fully. The rest period is necessary because this type of moxibustion has a slower, longer-acting effect than needling, and therefore time is required for the full results to manifest. I have also included a few key ideas from *Ken Sawada*'s moxibustion methods (which were developed before those of *Fukaya*), especially those concerning the movement of disease and therefore the order of moxibustion application.

Isaburo Fukaya's Ten Rules Of Moxibustion

1. The points have no inherent effects alone, but are made to be effective by the practitioner.

When disease occurs, points will become reactive (painful on pressure, hard, or concave); these points represent the keyholes through which the door to health can be opened. If the points are used properly, results that cannot be obtained using medication are achieved.

2. Descriptions of the points in the various texts give only a rough idea of their true location.

It is important initially to learn approximately where points are located, and then search for the clinically significant points on or near these points.

3. Points move according to the nature and progress of disease.

If patients are treated over a reasonable period of time, the use of moxa causes the points to disappear and/or move. For instance, when treating the upper thoracic area, the reactive points tend to disappear by moving upwards, almost as if the disease is being chased up and out of the body.

4. Try to understand and use famous/ well known points.

Rather than trying to use many extra points, it is far better to be able to use a few well known points effectively.

5. It is important to use as few points as possible to achieve a good result.

Where possible, it is best to use as few points as possible because nobody likes to be burned, no matter how skilfully, and too many points can produce a negative effect. Direct moxibustion provides a real chance to improve clinical skills because a mark remains at each point burned and causes the patient some discomfort. Therefore for the least discomfort with the maximum benefit it should be natural to be strict in point selection, thereby decreasing the number of points used. It is no accident that the best point locaters are normally those practitioners who are good at moxibustion.

6. Points that are not reactive yield poor results.

Points that may be appropriate theoretically, but are not valid in a given patient will produce no reaction. This means that the point is not appropriate for the patient at that time. By understanding the physiology and pathology of the patient and reading the pulse properly, the chances of finding the most appropriate points is improved. However, in the end they still have to be tested by the practitioner's fingers and thumbs to determine whether they are reactive.

7. It is not effective to treat only the location of the pain or the problem.

Treating the location of pain or a problem is not only ineffective but also impossible in some cases, for instance, eye pain, haemorrhoids, and toothache spring to mind. Even in cases where treating the location is possible, using additional points local or distal to the problem is more effective.

8. It is ineffective to rely solely on the fact that well-known points are being used.

Sometimes the most reactive point is not a well known point or even a regular point on a meridian. However, this is the point that should be used, not the well-known point, albeit nearby.

9. The size and number of cones should be adjusted according to the constitution of the patient.

For frail patients, it is advisable to lower the moxibustion dosage, whereas a stronger dosage is appropriate for stronger patients. The dosage can be thought of as being directly dependent on:

1. the number of points used;

2. the number of cones used on each point; and

3. the density of each cone, which is dependent on the hardness of rolling.

10. The points must be located skilfully.

If points are not located properly, they will not yield results. More time and care should be taken to find the most appropriate points than to treat the points.

ISABURO FUKAYA'S TREATMENT STRATEGY FOR ASTHMA

The following is a translation of *Isaburo Fukaya* 's treatment strategy for asthma, first presented in 1957 in Japan.

Asthma Treatment Strategy

I would like to present a few examples from my own record illustrating my approach to treating bronchial asthma. I use two steps in my treatment strategy, with the second step being carried out if the first step is ineffective.

The first step involves applying a large number of cones to *Zen Soku Yu*[47] (喘息兪) (see Figure 3-7), first mentioned by Mr. *Tamamori* in his *Shin Kyu Hi Bun* (鍼灸秘聞). *Zen Soku Yu* is located 3 *bu* (0.3 *cun*) above and lateral to *Kaku Yu* (膈兪; BL17) on the Bladder line. If this point is pressed with the ball of the thumb, a pleasant pain will be felt by asthma sufferers, in whom it is always reactive.

If the back is examined when an asthma attack is in progress, two bars of hardness will be found to run vertically on either side of the spine. Alternatively, a number of hard lumps on either side of the spine may be observed. This phenomenon is seen only when asthma is active. At times when this stiffness is not apparent, softening of these areas can remove the symptoms associated with asthma. This can usually be done by applying a large number of cones (30 to 50) to *Zen Soku Yu*.

Asthma sufferers vary widely, however, and the application of moxa only to *Zen Soku Yu* is sometimes insufficient to soften the stiff areas and produce relief of asthmatic symptoms. In these cases, the second step of the strategy is carried out. This

---

[47] *Zen Soku Yu* (喘息兪) could be translated as "Asthma *Shu* Point"

consists of finding the most painful points upon pressure to the upper back and shoulders. These points are most often found to be *Kin Shuku* (筋縮; GV8), *Shin Chu* (身柱; GV12), *Ken Sei* (肩井); GB21), *Ko Ko* (膏肓; BL43), *Hai Yu* (肺兪; BL13), *Shin Yu* (心兪; BL15), and *Ten Totsu* (天突; CV22) (Figure 3-7). Approximately seven half-rice grain- size cones should be applied to each of these points except *Kin Shuku*, to which many cones (30 to 50) should be applied. After the moxibustion has been applied, the points are checked again and if the stiffness has gone the treatment is finished.

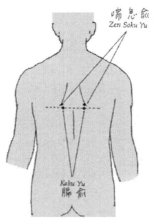

嘱息兪
Zen Soku Yu

Koku Yu
肺兪

Figure 3-8: Location of Zen Soku Yu
The point used in step 1 of *Isaburo Fukaya*'s asthma treatment strategy

For children, seven thread-size cones should be applied to *Zen Soku Yu* and *Shin Chu* as a basic treatment. After the symptoms have been quelled, I instruct the parents to apply moxa at home as a means of preventing further attacks. This should consist of five thread-size cones to each of these points every day for the first seven days of each month for an extended period. This often prevents any further attacks.

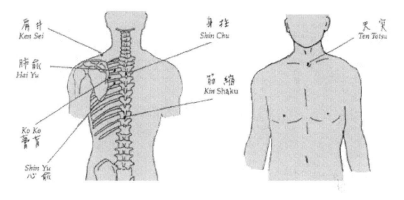

Figure 3-9: Location of the points used in step 2 of Isaburo Fukaya's asthma treatment strategy

Case History 1

History & Symptoms: A 51-year-old man, owner of a liquor store, initially presented on September 10, 1952. Symptoms consisted of severe cough and asthma. Inspection of the upper back and shoulders revealed stiff bars of hardness on either side of the spine on the upper back. The symptoms were more marked in winter.

Treatment: Step 1 treatment of *Zen Soku Yu,* was carried out. Fifty cones were applied to this point and there was no need to apply step 2.

After 10 consecutive days of moxibustion, the stiff areas began to soften and all asthma attacks were suppressed. Thereafter, for the first seven days of each month for one year, the above moxibustion treatment was carried out. There has been no subsequent recurrence of any asthmatic symptoms.

Case History 2

History & Symptoms: A 49-year-old housewife with little asthmatic coughing, but great difficulty in breathing first presented on November 5, 1953. The upper back and shoulders showed the characteristic bars of stiffness on either side of the spine. The symptoms were marked in winter.

Treatment: Applying 30 cones of moxa to *Zen Soku Yu* resulted in all symptoms disappearing. This was carried out for seven consecutive days. The second step was not needed. After the above treatments, the patient had more than three asthma attacks during the winter. Moxa was applied to *Zen Soku Yu* during each attack.

Case History 3

History & Symptoms: A 46-year-old male tailor had extremely severe coughing and asthmatic attacks whenever he became tired. The characteristic bars of stiffness were present in the upper back. Symptoms were marked in summer. Initial consultation was on June 10, 1954.

Treatment: Step 1 was carried out with 30 cones being burned on Zen Soku Yu for three consecutive days, but to no effect. The second step, involving burning 30 cones of moxa on *Kin Shuku* (GV8) and seven cones on the other points, was then carried out. Step 2 was continued for 10 consecutive days. Therefter asthma attacks recurred, but were treated effectively using the second- step moxibustion treatment.

Case History 4

History & Symptoms: A 50-year old male pharmacist was prone to asthma attacks in the winter and would take medication. Coughing was particularly severe, and the characteristic upper back and shoulder stiffness was present. Initial consultation was August 5, 1954.

Treatment: Step 1 and step 2 were carried out. Step 1 was carried out at the time of an attack for two consecutive days, but with unsatisfactory results. Step 2 was implemented, but also with unsatisfactory results. The treatments were terminated at this point.

Case History 5

History & Symptoms: A 6-year-old boy had severe coughing and asthma that was marked in winter. The upper back had scattered, stiff areas. Initial consultation was on October 5, 1953.

Treatment: Seven thread-size cones of moxa were applied to *Zen Soku Yu* and also to *Shin Chu* (CV12). This caused the symptoms to disappear. The above treatment was carried out once at the beginning of each month for one year. There have been no subsequent recurrences.

Comment

Examining the treatments, one should be struck by their simplicity: moxibustion was the only modality used. Also, *Fukaya*'s determination and faith in moxibustion are evident. To choose just two points, the left and right *Zen Soku Yu*, and work with a patient who is having difficulty breathing requires a strong belief in the efficacy of what you are doing. This comes with study and experience, and through palpating the points properly, which gives the patient and the practitioner a sensory taste of the potential of the point for healing. This allows the patient to bear 50 or more cones and the practitioner can tell whether he's on to a winner. On a physical level, the points should be palpated regularly (maybe every 15 cones) to assess whether the tissues have relaxed and whether more cones are needed. It should be noted that the points mentioned by *Fukaya* are usually hard and painful upon pressure in asthmatic patients, which would allow dispersive moxibustion (hard rolled cones or a large number of cones) to be burnt without excessive pain. This is probably suitable for deficient heat in the Lungs.

Another clue to the progress of treatment is whether the skin around the points becomes red. The patient can also confirm whether there are any changes in sensation with moxibustion. For instance, if heat is initially not felt very strongly, one method is to continue applying cones until heat is no longer felt. In most of the case histories described above, the worsening of symptoms in winter and the stiffness in the upper back and shoulders would indicate that the patients probably have Kidney deficiency syndromes. Many people in post-World War II were malnourished, nervous, and fighting for survival, and therefore Kidney *Yin* deficiency is a definite possibility. The results obtained with moxibustion under such harsh conditions bear testimony to its effectiveness. In today's prosperous well-nourished society, moxibustion should be even more effective.

The final point to note is that the systematic treatment pattern ensures that asthma does not recur.

KEN SAWADA'S BUDDHIST GAMMADION (SWASTIKA)

The Buddhist 卐 symbol has great meaning and symbolism that are applicable to treatment. *Sawada* believed that the Christian cross symbol was theoretically good, but lacked the practical refinement of the Buddhist symbol. He applied this symbol to the human body, with its centre at the navel; the movement of *Ki* is shown by the arms of the symbol (Figure 3-9). The left side (*Yang*) has a tendency to sink and the right side (*Yin*) has a tendency to rise; the left side rotates to the right at the bottom and the right rotates to the left at the top. Four points known as the *Four Spirits* (四靈),comprising the left and right *Katsu Niku Mon* (滑肉門; ST24) and the left and right *Dai Ko* (大巨; ST27) are of particular note in this grid.

For problems affecting the right lower abdomen, the left lower abdomen would be treated; for problems affecting the upper right abdomen, the lower right abdomen would be treated. In addition, problems affecting the upper right abdomen appear on the upper left part of the abdomen.

Diagonal considerations can also be made; for instance, pain upon pressure at the right *Ki Mon* (期門; LV14) can be relieved by needling the left *Dai Ko* (ST27) and pain at the left *Ki Mon* (LV14) can be relieved by needling the right DaiKo (ST27).

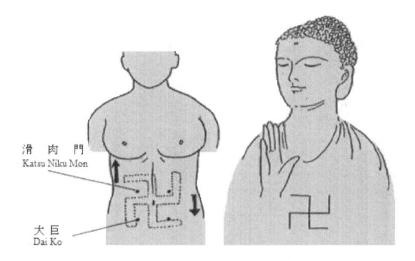

Figure 3-10: Illustration showing Ken Sawada's application of the Buddhist Gammadion symbol to treatment.

The Four Spirits

The left and right *Katsu Niku Mon* and *Dai Ko* were given the name "the Four Spirits" by *Ken Sawada*. He explained that "Cold *Ki* from heaven enters the body through *Fu Mon* (風門; BL12) and proceeds into the diaphragm, Liver, Spleen, and Kidneys, at which time it appears at *Katsu Niku Mon* (ST24). *Katsu Niku Mon* is the most effective point for removing cold pathogen that has entered the internal organs. The point can be treated with both moxa and needling. Tonsillitis, middle ear infections, and inflammation of the parotid gland can be cured in one treatment using this point. It is a curious thing. Needling can be carried out up to a depth of 1.5 to 2 cun with no problem."

The other "two spirits," *Dai Ko* (ST27), are explained as follows: "The cold *Ki* from the earth enters *San In Ko* (三陰交; SP6), goes into the Stomach, and then descends to *Dai Ko*. If it (the cold *Ki*) is then expelled through diarrhoea, there will not be a problem; however, if it is not expelled, it collects at the *Mu* point of the Large Intestine, *Ten Su* (天枢; ST25), and causes swelling. This is (manifests as) intestinal typhoid. In dysentery, this cold *Ki* collects in the Small Intestine and is less serious than typhoid. The lower *Ki* (from the earth) goes to the Large Intestine and appears at *Dai Ko*. The most effective point for removing earth *Ki* from the Large Intestine is *Dai Ko*. From *Dai Ko* the earth *Ki* can go upwards to *Ki Mon* (LV14), entering the Lungs and pleural cavity. Thus it can be seen that *Dai Ko* is the starting point for pneumonia and pleurisy. Pneumonia and pleurisy are the result of cold rising up and penetrating into the body. This causes *Ki* and blood to move contrary to their normal healthy direction (逆). This (upward movement of cold *Ki*) is the cause of this problem.

The Four Spirits can correct this reversal. *Dai Ko* can be used very effectively for intestinal problems, including diarrhoea, constipation, and intestinal catarrh as well as for bronchial catarrh, throat catarrh, pneumonia, and pleurisy. It is also very effective for diseases of the uterus, excessive vaginal discharge, and menstrual problems. Menstrual problems (most) come from chilling of the uterus and the blood vessels, causing them to become constricted."

Comment

Sawada's ideas are a beacon, particularly in the way that he combines traditional theory with his own observations. In my own practice, I have helped someone with right shoulder problems by loosening up the lower right abdomen. I find that the lower right abdomen is often problematic due to complications related to chronic and acute inflammation of the appendix and the after effects of surgery (appendectomy). In the old texts, this area is the place where chronic cold (久寒) is said to collect and cause stiffness. Whether *Sawada* was aware of this chronic cold location is not known.

The lower right abdomen also causes problems with the right ribcage. I have often found that a person with a Spleen deficient disposition affected by a cold or influenza readily shows pain and stiffness at *Katsu Niku Mon*.

The idea of cold coming in through *San In Ko (SP6)* from the earth is also very interesting because *Kyu To Shin* (moxa head needling) to this point is one of the best ways of warming up the lower abdomen and I use it frequently.

CHAPTER 4

Posture and Being Relaxed

4.1   STANDING AT A FUNERAL

EO: "You look like you are standing at a funeral. Why are you doing that?" *(said with a puzzled look)*

TS: Well – I'm doing the standing[48]. I thought that this was a good approach to treatment... ...to allow the *Ki* to flow well..."

EO: You need to understand the difference between practice and treatment. Now I understand why it feels like you are at a funeral – the standing is for you – it's your time – it's introspective and you gather *Ki* to yourself. In treatment you have to connect – communicate – let your *Ki* flow out – it is all about the patient and you forget yourself completely.

---

[48] Standing refers to the *I Chuan* system of standing meditation as taught by Master Sam Tam.

TS: Ok – but I'm sure I see you doing it too from time to time, *Sensei* – you pause when needling and sink your *Ki* – I can see it and feel it.

EO: Yes – it's true – now and then I do – it happens – when I need to focus or for other reasons – but only then.

TS: But I find that if I stand all day without doing it then my lower back starts to lock-up.

EO: You do the standing practice to get strength and build capability in all positions – do you think that *Sifu* is always in the standing position when he does his art – no – his practice allows him to know his position even when he is in the natural position which he finds himself in. You do the standing to improve your *Ki* so you can be yourself when you need to be. Be yourself – it's not so bad you know – Just be yourself.

4.2   *OSHIDE* (押し手)

GW: Last week you needled a patient using an unorthodox left hand (押し手; *oshide*) position and I asked why. You then asked me what the functions of the *oshide* were. I thought that one function was to send or receive *Ki* to and from the patient. Another was for stability.

EO: Yes they are right. Then once the person can do those things, then the *oshide* shape becomes less important. As long as you can fulfill those functions, then that's OK. The shape isn't everything For example, people don't primarily buy cars because of their design, speed etc. The primary purpose is to get from A to B. Of course, in order to travel faster, the shape of the car must change slightly i.e. less wind resistance. To carry 100 people you will again need a different style of car. The purpose influences the shape… not the other way round.

If you go to some study groups there will no doubt be some people who try to use the same *oshide* for the nose as for the back. Always. Then there'll be another type who say "I'm now using one of *Sugiyama's* 18 *oshide!*". However, the main thing here is whether the *oshide* being used is suitable for the area being treated now, whether the shape is suitable for the purpose you want to achieve. There are not only 18 types, there are thousands.

The particular shape or type isn't important. The purpose and the fact that the *oshide* matches that purpose is. If you are able to answer the question as to what the purpose of the *oshide* is, then that means that your *oshide* can adjust to many different situations and purposes at various times. But, if you forget or lose the purpose when treating, then obviously your *oshide* will become very rigid.

There are a vast array of possible *oshide,* yet to define them under just 18 shapes and say these shapes are good and all others aren't, is rubbish. In early times when acupuncturists worked, there was no book compiled of 18 *oshide* was there? Those people used different *oshide* gleaned from their experience. Beginners would see the different *oshide* being used, but without the necessary experience, they use them incorrectly.

GW: When needling the buttock, say... ...the buttock on the other side to where I'm standing, I want make sure my *oshide* is strong and steady first of all. After getting stable, then I want to needle from a little way in. I find that this requires a considerable amount of strength. By trying to maintain this shape, I find my back and arms becoming tense. I know the *Ki* isn't flowing when I'm like this.

EO: I can show you by example. If I just try to use my arms to pull you down, then it requires a lot of effort and actually it gets me little effect. But, I can do it much more effectively by not just relying on my arms alone. It's the same with massage. Instead of forcing the pressure, you just rest on it to get the same effect. Do the *oshide* with that same way of thinking. It's exactly as *Sifu* was saying. I don't want you to think that to use the body to create the *oshide* means to lean into it.

Don't use force. If need be, go around the bed and needle from the other side! If you feel tired after a days work, you must analyze how you do things and find where you are doing it wrong.

It's true that as long as you do something in the correct position and posture, no matter what the work is, you can do it. The workload is spread throughout the whole body. This way, the body can work much more than you expect. We have to learn this. It's a feeling of being very light and a feeling where you aren't using any strength. If you can do it this way, then obviously the *Ki* will flow too.

4.3   RELAX FROM TENSION

We have to keep the patient comfortable so that they can relax. Then we can do something. Really if possible we should have a position which is comfortable for both the practitioner and the patient to give a good treatment. In the case of this patient however I am deliberately making the muscle tight so that is exposes the underlying tension – in this case of the 胆経 (Gallbladder meridian). This is different. You see in oriental medicine it is this... ...*and* that... ...*and* something else all at the same time. Now for him, that Gallbladder channel has always been troublesome. So I want to loosen from the starting point of being in a tense position. If I can loosen it even just a little in the tensed position, then in the relaxed position it will be a lot better. You see it is difficult to relax someone *more* when they already feel that they are relaxed.

- *A Long Road* continues in Volume II

A LONG ROAD

Made in the USA
San Bernardino, CA
21 December 2016